Liver Cancer - Genesis, Progression and Metastasis

Edited by Mark Feitelson and Alla Arzumanyan

Published in London, United Kingdom

Liver Cancer - Genesis, Progression and Metastasis
http://dx.doi.org/10.5772/intechopen.100845
Edited by Mark Feitelson and Alla Arzumanyan

Contributors
Muhammad Aqib, Muhammad Usman, Aqsa Nazir, S.S. Haque, Mehboobus Salam, Ravi Bhushan Raman, Anna Rossetto, Alessandro Uzzau, Alessandro Rosignoli, Brunilda Tatani, Valli De Re, Alisa Petkevich, Aleksandr Abramov, Vadim Pospelov, Shihai Liu, Kai Sun, Maen A. Abdelrahim, Alan Hodges, Cheng Jin, Bo-Shi Wang, You-Yi Liu

First published in London, United Kingdom, 2023 by IntechOpen
IntechOpen is the global imprint of INTECHOPEN LIMITED, registered in England and Wales, registration number: 11086078, 5 Princes Gate Court, London, SW7 2QJ, United Kingdom

British Library Cataloguing-in-Publication Data
A catalogue record for this book is available from the British Library

Additional hard and PDF copies can be obtained from orders@intechopen.com

Liver Cancer - Genesis, Progression and Metastasis
Edited by Mark Feitelson and Alla Arzumanyan
p. cm.
Print ISBN 978-1-80356-413-5
Online ISBN 978-1-80356-414-2
eBook (PDF) ISBN 978-1-80356-415-9

Meet the editors

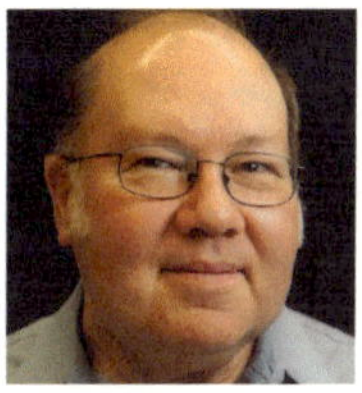

Mark Feitelson received his Ph.D. in Microbiology and Immunology from UCLA in 1979. He began his work on the pathogenesis of chronic hepatitis B at Stanford University and was then recruited to the Fox Chase Cancer Center by Nobel laureate Dr. Baruch Blumberg. In 1991, Dr. Feitelson moved to Thomas Jefferson University where he became a Professor of Pathology and Cell Biology and director of the Molecular Diagnostics Lab in Microbiology. In 2007, Dr. Feitelson was appointed Professor of Biology at Temple University. He is also the CSO of SFA Therapeutics. His work has been supported by NIH, industry and foundations, and he has mentored over 130 students. He has more than 150 publications, 180 abstracts and 11 patents.

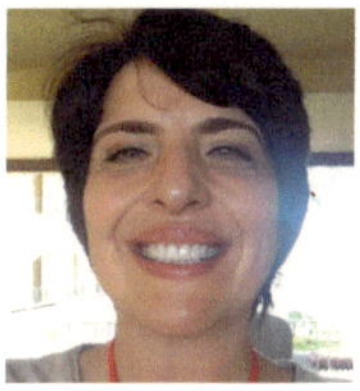

Alla Arzumanyan received her Ph.D. in Biotechnology from Yerevan State University, Armenia in 2003. She pursued postdoctoral training at Temple University and Thomas Jefferson University in Philadelphia, USA. In 2008 she joined Dr. Feitelson's group and is currently a Research Associate Professor. She has worked on the pathogenesis of hepatitis B and has developed an artificial immune system to diagnose serious human pathogens. She is Chief Development Officer for SFA Therapeutics and has developed a novel microbiome-based treatment for plaque psoriasis. She has co-authored 17 original papers and three book chapters, and has presented 17 posters/invited talks.

Contents

Preface

Hepatocellular cancer (HCC) is among the ten most common tumor types worldwide. It is associated with chronic hepatitis B and C virus infections, chronic alcoholism, and with nonalcoholic steatohepatitis (NASH). HCC most often develops against a background of chronic liver disease (CLD), in which hepatitis progressively develops into fibrosis, cirrhosis, and finally cancer. This suggests that regardless of etiology, the pathogenesis of HCC is immune-mediated. Early-stage HCC is usually asymptomatic, and in most cases, by the time diagnosis is made, HCC is often in advanced stages, resulting in high mortality. A major limitation in achieving an early diagnosis, as well as developing and assessing the efficacy of therapeutics targeting HCC, is the lack of reproducible biomarkers. Major efforts are underway to develop such markers as an understanding of the molecular pathogenesis of HCC increases. Given that HCC, like most other tumor types, is a multi-step process, it has been challenging to develop effective therapeutics. A variety of local and systemic therapies are currently in use to treat HCC, but the patient response rate is modest. However, the renin-angiotensin system, insulin resistance, cancer stem cells, and specific epigenetic changes in hepatocellular gene expression are putative targets for the development of new therapies. Altered expression patterns of miRNAs may also contribute to the pathogenesis of HCC and serve as therapeutic targets. Dysbiosis of the gut microbiome, which is characterized by alterations in the ratios of microbes in the intestine, may also mediate alterations in gene expression in hepatocytes and immune cells that are important to the pathogenesis of CLD. However, it is not always clear whether altered patterns of gene expression mediate HCC development or reflect the outcome of tumorigenesis. The HCC microenvironment is also characteristically tolerogenic, which attenuates the efficacy of newer treatments, such as cancer immunotherapy. The application of immunotherapy and/or the resolution of dysbiosis prior to the development of cancer may also be a viable option to alter the progression of CLD. The tumor microenvironment is also altered by changes in glucose metabolism in which oxidative metabolism is replaced by aerobic glycolysis in tumor cells. Future research will determine whether the biological properties of tumor cells, the tumor microenvironment, the gut microbiome, and/or immune effector cells will be the best target in developing more effective therapies against HCC.

Mark Feitelson
Department of Biology,
Temple University,
Philadelphia, PA, USA

Alla Arzumanyan
Temple University,
Philadelphia, PA, USA

Chapter 1

Etiology, Mechanism and Treatment of Liver Cancer

Aqsa Nazir, Muhammad Aqib and Muhammad Usman

Abstract

Liver cancer or hepatocellular carcinoma (HCC) is a malignant tumor in liver tissue and worldwide it is fourth leading death cause among all cancers. The most common causes of liver cancer are hepatitis B or C virus infections, alcoholic liver disease (ALD), nonalcoholic fatty liver disease (NAFLD) to non-alcoholic steatohepatitis (NASH), smoking and obesity. The development and metastasis of liver cancer is a multistage and branched process of morphological and genetic traits. Various corresponding signaling pathways such as Yes-Associated Protein-Hippo Pathway (YAP-HIPPO), Wnt/β-catenin and inflammation by interleukin-6 (IL-6), tumor necrosis factor (TNF), nuclear factor-Kb (NF-κB), biological pathways including epithelial–mesenchymal transition (EMT), tumor microenvironment, tumor-stromal interactions and cancer stem cells and gut microbial dysbiosis are allied to both origination, progression and metastasis of liver cancer. Numerous therapeutic approaches are classified into different categories such as pharmacological therapy including sorafenib, lenvatinib and ramuciruma, surgery of HCC patients includes surgical resection, adjuvant therapy after surgical resection and liver transplantation. Loco-regional ablative therapy includes cryotherapy, ethanol injection and radiofrequency ablation, cytotoxic chemotherapy, natural compounds such as piperine, as curcumin and oleocanthal, oncolytic virus therapy, immunotherapies and nanotechnology.

Keywords: hepatocellular carcinoma (HCC), inflammation, disease progression, Dysbiosis, hepatitis B and C

1. Introduction

Liver cancer is a malignant tumor which is commonly occurs in cirrhosis and chronic liver disease patients. Liver cancer comprises of different types, the most common type is hepatocellular carcinoma (HCC) or primary liver cancer and other rarely occurring types includes hepatoblastoma and intrahepatic cholangiocarcinoma depend upon their origin such as liver stem cells, hepatocytes, cholangiocytes, and hepatoblasts [1]. Worldwide, the fourth leading cause of all cancers related deaths is primary liver cancer or HCC and its prevalence is 75% of all types of liver cancers. Out of all types of cancer related patients, every fifth male and seventh in female is diagnosed with liver cancer. Moreover, World Health Organization (WHO) declared that if it is not properly treated then ultimately in 2030 more than one million individuals will die from this ailment [2].

The liver cancer is most prevalent in Middle and Western Africa and East and Southeast Asia countries, whereas lowest ratio was found in Northern and Eastern Europe and South-Central and Western Asia. The variation in prevalence of liver cancer in different regions is due to diverse exposure to hepatitis viruses and other environmental pathogens. As in developing countries, 60% infection is caused by hepatitis B virus (HBV) and 33% infection is caused by hepatitis C virus (HCV) of total liver cancer. Currently, in United States and Central Europe, liver cancer prevalence and mortality is also increased to an alarming situation as more than 750,000 new cases annually, because of high HCV by regular drug use and nonalcoholic fatty liver disease by obesity epidemic, or might be due to alcohol-related cirrhosis. In spite of the advancement, liver cancer is still one of the most challenging cancer to treat. The clinical output remains low and about one-third patients eligible to curative approaches of HCC such as local destructive therapies, surgery and liver transplantation. The surgical removal is possible in 5–15% of patients in early stages, without cirrhosis and due to reduced hepatic restoration capacity in later stages. Therefore, the survival rate can be increased by early diagnosis and application of curative approaches. In early HCC treatment the five-year survival rate is 47–53%, which is still not satisfactory. However, the chances of recurrence of HCC remain high even after curative treatment [3].

2. Risk factors

The most common etiological risk factors of liver cancer are hepatitis B or C virus infections, alcoholic liver disease (ALD), nonalcoholic fatty liver disease (NAFLD) to non-alcoholic steatohepatitis (NASH) and chronic alcohol consumption, although smoking, obesity, iron overload and diabetes are also associated with liver cancer [4]. Worldwide about 80% of HCC is allied to chronic infections of hepatitis B and C viruses, as hepatitis B virus is responsible more than the hepatitis C virus. About 10–25% HCC or cirrhosis deaths cause by hepatitis B viruses and it mainly affect in early age of life. The vaccine for hepatitis B marketed in 1982, have been targeted to newborns. In 2017, about 187 WHO member countries vaccinated the newborns and globally 84% population received three doses of hepatitis B vaccine. However, hepatitis C virus rarely affect children, and only 15–45% patients recovered from this and remaining people lead to chronic infection of liver. It is asymptomatic, and for many years, chronic infections not clinically evident [5].

Alcohol and smoking are major contributor to liver cancer. The USA studies showed that light-to-moderate alcohol consumption which is less than three drinks per day significantly reduced HCC risk [6]. The alcohol consumption is more in high societies as compared to low income regions, while smoking ratio is high in middle and low income regions as compared to high income countries. A report in 2014 found that cigarette smoking at that time was linked with a 70% high risk of liver cancer, while 40% in previous years [7]. Obesity cause low grade inflammation, leads to metabolic dysfunction, development of NAFLD to NASH, cirrhosis, fibrosis and in turn liver cancer. Research claimed that overweight and obesity cause 18% and 83% high risks of liver cancer and the HCC risk twice with the diabetes disease [5].

Some other risk factors of liver cancer are congenital abnormalities, toxic aflatoxin or arsenic contaminated food and autoimmune liver diseases. The congenital abnormalities include hemochromatosis, Wilson's disease, alpha-1-antitrypsin deficiency and hereditary tyrosinemia. However, the aflatoxins are released by the fungi such as

Aspergillus parasiticus and *Aspergillus flavus* in contaminated food. The autoimmune hepatitis is also a cause of liver cirrhosis and HCC but the chances of occurrence is far less than the hepatitis B and C viruses [8–10]. All these risk factors are cumulative and influence each other such as if a person is suffering with hepatitits B or C and consume alcohol then he will be at severe risk of the pathogenesis of HCC by the interplay of environmental, viral, diet and host factors. These factors develop chronic liver disease which may lead to liver cirrhosis by numerous mutagens for example oxidative stress, chemical exposure and deviation in the DNA repair leads to genome alteration which ultimately results in cancerous genome in which chronic inflammation, reactive oxygen and nitrogen species, and mutation are the main aspects of hepatocytes necrosis.

3. Progression and metastasis of HCC

The main mechanism in the development of liver cancer is the inflammation in liver, except the cause of it. The inflammation is the automatic immune response to the targeted cells, which leads to hepatic necrosis. In early stages the inflammatory signaling pathway is activated by reactive oxygen species (ROS) and nitric oxide (NO), which produce chemokines, prostaglandins, cytokines, growth factors and proangiogenic factors, that transforms the hepatocytes and cause initiation of anti-apoptotic processing and restriction of immune surveillance and develop liver fibrosis and in later stages the liver tissue damaged permanently, called liver cirrhosis. More than 80% of primary liver cancer is caused by the chronic liver diseases commonly appear on a background of liver cirrhosis. If it persists and not treated it will metastasis to other liver tissues and diagnosed as liver cancer or HCC, causing morbidity and the mortality (**Figure 1**) [12, 13].

3.1 Signaling pathways

The development of liver cancer is a multistage and branched process of morphological and genetic traits. The tumor in liver is not only associated with cellular malignancy but also linked with genome abnormality, which ultimately cause neoplastic growth. In HCC, frequently mutation occurs in cell cycle genes i.e. CDKN2A (cyclin-dependent kinase inhibitor 2A) and CCND1 (encodes cyclin D1) and cancer gens such as WNT, TP53, and CTNNB1(encodes βcatenin). The hepatic-carcinogenesis emerged by two most important oncogenic events such as telomerase reverse transcriptase (TERT) activation and MYC activation. These genes activated in various forms of liver tumors. The TERT activation is required for

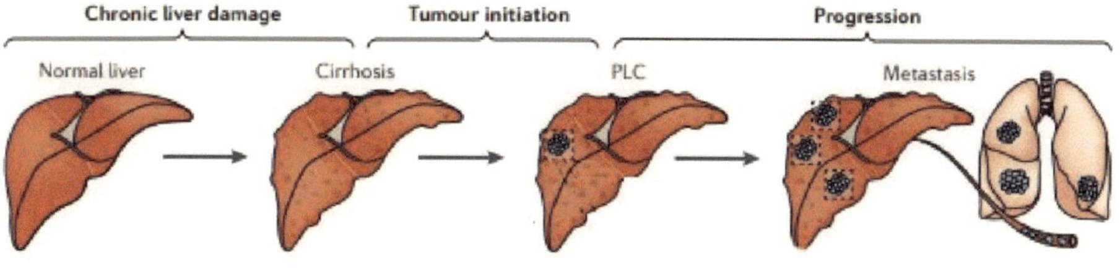

Figure 1.
Progression and metastasis of liver cancer [11].

unlimited proliferation and MYC activate for transformation of normal liver cells into HCC at later stage of cancer [11, 14]. Along with genetics, the epigenetics also play a vital role to the pathogenesis of cancer. The epigenetic alterations include DNA hypo-methylation or hyper-methylation, chromatin remodeling, dysregulation of histone adaptation patterns, aberrant expression of micro-RNAs (miRNAs) and long noncoding RNAs (lncRNAs) are allied with HCC. As in hepatitis B, the HBx protein constitutively activates the pathways in **Figure 2**. The epigenetic alteration patterns can affect the frequencies and types of genetic modifications at the adjacent chromatin regions and some of the genetic mutations in HCC regulate epigenetic changes in host gene expression. Therefore, both factors appear to be inseparable and promote tumorigenesis synergistically.

Researchers are trying from decades to reveal the molecular mechanisms of cancer origination and progression. Conversely, the heterogeneity and diverse characteristics of cancer commonly cause confusion. Nowadays, it is widely recognized that cancer develops from normal cells to malignant stages in many years because of its multistep process. The cells become tumorigenic and show malignant phenotypes due to numerous hallmarks. Same as for other solid tumors, the HCC is also described with those cancer hallmarks for example evading growth suppressors, sustained cell proliferation, cell death resistance, metastasis, invasion, angiogenesis, and deregulated energy metabolism. These hallmarks and genetic or epigenetic alterations linkage helps to recognize the molecular mechanisms. However, various corresponding signaling pathways are allied to both origination and progression of liver cancer. These mechanisms include Yes-Associated Protein-Hippo Pathway (YAP-HIPPO), Wnt/β-catenin and inflammation by interleukin-6 (IL-6), tumor necrosis factor (TNF), nuclear factor-Kb (NF-κB). Moreover, PPARγ induced lipid metabolism, epigenetic alterations like acetylation of histones, DNA methylation, and noncoding RNAs also cause progression and metastasis of HCC [11, 15].

Hippo-YAP pathway control the size, multiplication, apoptosis, and invasion of hepatic cells by YAZ-HIPPO receptors, which regulate the YAZ/TAZ transcriptional genes. WNT/AXIN controls the β-catenin protein transfer to the nucleus, forming the YAZ/TAZ-β-catenin-TCF trimer, which stimulate TGF-β as a profibrotic agent and C-Myc as a proliferative agent, cause cancer initiation, proliferation, progression, resistance to anticancerous drugs [16, 17]. The NF – κB is inhibited by IκB protein, when IκB is phosphorylated by kinase complex (IKK) into in Ser32 and Ser36, IκB is degraded by proteasomal complex and translocate NF – κB P50/P65 which mainly involved in apoptosis inhibition, tumor cell proliferation, progression, cancer initiation and drug resistance. PPARγ at one side inhibit the β-catenin and NF-κB signaling pathways by bonding to its ligands, on the other side it is involved in apoptosis, inhibition of cell proliferation, and metastasis by binding to the peroxisome proliferating response elements (PPRE) which act as specific response elements in nucleus [18, 19]. These signaling pathways upregulate or downregulate according to etiological factors of HCC. For example, Hepatitis B is a DNA virus and it incorporate into host by various ways such as hijack its machinery, oxidative stress, and Hepatitis B protein x. Hepatitis B activate TERT, Cyclin A2, PDGFR, EGFR gene expressions. Hepatitis B protein x stimulates Wnt/β-catenin, NFB, TGF-β, P53 and ROS signaling pathways for the pathogenesis of HCC. While hepatitis C is a RNA virus and it induce inflammation by release of pro-inflammatory cytokines such as IL-6, TNF-α, IL-1 and IL-18, modify TGF-β signaling pathway and glucose and lipid metabolism for the HCC development. Similarly, chronic alcohol consumption activates cytochrome CYP2E1 and cause liver steatosis and inflammation which leads to HCC.

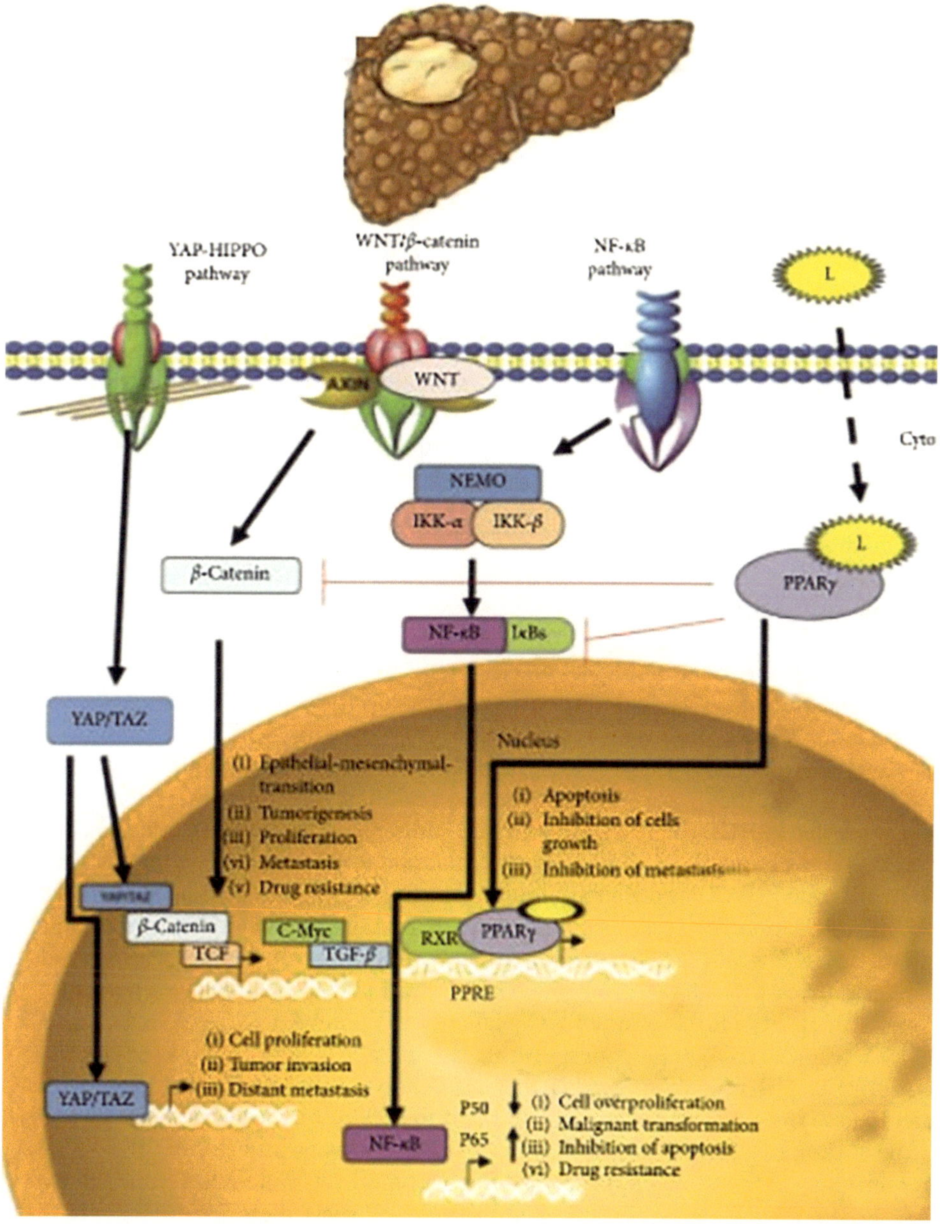

Figure 2.
Different signal pathway of HCC progression.

Histone modification is carried out by enzymes which add or remove acetyl groups with histones. The de-acetylation of histone proteins by histone acetyltransferase (HAT) enzyme leads to malignant proliferation, transformation, and invasion of tumor cells. The DNA methylation is common in liver cancer and 3000 hypo-methylated promoters were identified in HCC tumor, one of them is CpG methylation which is controlled by DNA methyltransferases (DNMTs) enzyme. The DNMTs also methylated the genes like p16, p15, E-cadherin, hyper-methylated in cancer 1

(HIC-1), and Ras association domain family 1 isoform A (RASSF1A), which involved in cell adhesion, mobility, proliferation and invasion. The microRNAs (miRNAs) dysregulation causes abnormal gene expressions, leads to development, invasion, and metastasis of tumor cells. The main two miRNAs which contribute to HCC development are miR-122 and miR-221. In miR-122 liver become inflammed, steatohepatitis, and fibrosis occurs, whereas in miR-221 cellular pathways modulated, specifically linked to cell proliferation, survival, and metastasis [20–22]. Hepatitis B protein x blocks expression of E-cadherin and activates histone deacetylases 1 and 2. Hepatitis B protein x also affects expression of several miRNAs, which are also important in maintaining hepatitis C virus replication, persistence and progression of chronic liver disease to HCC. Hepatitis B and alcohol both involved in DNA methylation proliferate hepatocytes and eventually cause HCC. Hepatitis C virus core protein and the E2 envelope protein stimulate cell growth in liver cancer by lipid peroxidation and a mitochondrial dysfunction with oxidative stress. The hepatitis C core protein also alter gene expression and intracellular regulation mechanisms. Moreover, the hepatitis C virus non-structural 5A protein interacts with beta-catenin and stimulates its transcriptional activity in a phosphoinositide-3 kinase-dependent fashion to promote HCC pathogenesis.

3.2 Biological pathways

There are some other biological mechanisms which also play a vital role in progression of HCC such as epithelial–mesenchymal transition (EMT), tumor microenvironment, tumor-stromal interactions and cancer stem cells. In EMT process, epithelial cells drop their adhesive properties, which allow the mesenchymal membrane to migrate the cells, that grabbed by cancer cells and increase their dissemination all over the body. In HCC the EMT effectors i.e. cadherins, vimentin, fibronectin and integrins transformed and allow mesenchymal phenotype easily. The transcriptional factors like Slug, Twist and Zeb upregulated in supporting EMT pathway during HCC progression. Moreover, tumor-stromal interactions also promote HCC development, as hepatic stellate cells (HSCs) accumulate by the stimulation of hypoxia-induced platelet-derived growth factor-BB (PDGF-BB) and multiply in the tumor stroma along with upsurge in vascular endothelial growth factor-A (VEGF-A) expression in HSCs result in HCC angiogenesis. Similarly, signal transducer and activator of transcription (STAT3) act as a mediator between liver cancer cells and stromal cells interactions and regulate micro-environment for tumor formation [9, 23]. Alcohol consumption, hepatitis B and C all promote EMT pathway, and tumor micro-environment is also affected by hypoxia and hypoxia might stimulate EMT and the liver fibrosis and cirrhosis is highly activated by HSCs, all these factors contribute to the progression of HCC.

The cancer stem cell (CSC) also involved in progression, aggressiveness and metastasis of HCC, by the action of several surface markers such as epithelial cell adhesion molecule (EpCAM), CD13, CD44, CD90 and CD133. The acquisition of liver CSC in tumor cells caused by dedifferentiation and reprogramming of non-CSCs such as hepatoblasts, biliary cells and mature hepatocytes. For example, Sal-like protein 4 (SALL4) is a proto-oncogene in liver and embryonic stem cells and cause HCCC progression. The investigation proved that CSCs are considered to be more tumorigenic than non-stem cancer cells and they are resistant to numerous anticancer treatments, including chemotherapy and radiotherapy [24, 25]. The metabolic stress such as obesity and diabetes promotes Various evident studies show the signaling pathways, their functional process and tumor features as descried in **Table 1**. Hepatitis B protein x promotes the development of stemness characteristics in liver cells, which is part of the mechanism whereby hepatitis B protein x contributes to hepato-carcinogenesis. The long-term inflammation by hepatitis B or C virus, chronic alcohol consumption or and NASH, highly contribute to reprogramming of non-CSC into CSCs.

3.3 Gut microbial dysbiosis

The gut-liver axis is a dual anatomical and functional interaction between and gastrointestinal tract mainly by portal vein blood circulation. The synergetic relationship between liver and gut microbiota is regulated by a complex network of interactions, comprises of neuroendocrine, immune, and metabolic systems. There is a tight junction within the gut epithelium which act as a natural barrier to bacteria and their metabolic products. There is evidence that the gut microbiota moves beyond the gut by intestinal dysbiosis, which involved in hepatic carcinoma progression. Dysbiosis is a process in which tight junction of proteins disrupt and gut mucous layer become thinner, which leads to dysfunctional intestinal barrier. Particularly, dysbiosis stimulate the release of cancer-promoting metabolites, like secondary bile acids which consist of deoxycholic acid (DCA). Dysbiosis is also commonly associated with decreased levels of bacteria that produce the anti-inflammatory and anti-tumorigenic metabolites, short chain fatty acids. The dysfunctional gut barrier in dysbiosis increase intestinal permeability, bacterial overgrowth, bacterial translocation and immune system dysplasia, which results in leaky gut. The gut microbial dysbiosis deteriorates

Functional process	Signaling pathway	Phenotypic and tumor features	References
Cell cycle	p53 and RB–E2F	Aggressive phenotype and loss of DNA damage repair mechanisms	[26]
Development and differentiation	WNT–β-catenin	Activation in tumor-initiating cells (early and late stages)	
	SALL4	Poor prognosis and activation in tumor-initiating cells	[27]
	NF2	Stem cell features and tumor initiation	
Proliferation and survival	EGFR	Aggressive phenotype and reprogramming	[28]
	IGF	Pre-neoplastic lesions (early stage)	
Immune response	IL-6 signaling	Progenitor-derived response to adjuvant interferon therapy	[29]
	NF-κB	Chronic inflammation	
Angiogenesis	PDGF	Liver cirrhosis	[27]
	VEGF	Aggressive phenotype, poor prognosis and metastasis	
Stress response	ROS, NO	Oxidative phosphorylation (late stage)	[26]

EGFR, epidermal growth factor receptor; IGF, insulin-like growth factor; IL, interleukin; IL-6R, IL-6 receptor; NF2, neurofibromin 2; NF-κB, nuclear factor-κB; PDGF, platelet-derived growth factor; ROS, reactive oxygen species; SALL4, Sal-like protein 4; VEGF, vascular endothelial growth factor.

Table 1.
Major functional processes and signaling pathways in HCC development.

the metabolism, nutrition, immunity and inflammatory status of the liver. Numerous bacteria's such as *Streptococcus*, *Lactobacillus*, *Escherichia Shigella* and *Bacteroides* move into the portal vein and liver, which stimulates hepatic kupffer cells and stellate cells. They release a series of inflammatory mediators, increase levels of endotoxin, blood ammonia, provoke intestinal mucosal damage, stimulate liver cell steatosis and chronic inflammation, which cause the development of hepatic encephalopathy, liver fibrosis, cirrhosis and eventually leads to development of HCC [30].

Moreover, on the other hand, these liver diseases worse the gut microbial dysbiosis, as liver cirrhosis decreases gastric acid and bile acid secretion, function of lipopolysaccharide, bacteria, metabolites, and bowel movement, both leads to the overgrowth of intestinal bacteria and gut microbial dysbiosis.by affecting the stability and function of the gut microbiota. The gut microbiota of hepatic disorders such as hepatitis B and C viruses, ALD, NAFLD, NASH and HCC is significantly different from healthy microbiota such as amount of microbiota, species present, and metabolites produced due to gut microbial dysbiosis. For instance, in hepatitis B cirrhosis Faecalibacterium prausnitzii, and Enterococcus faecalis significantly increased, whereas *Bifidobacteria* and *Lactobacillus* significantly reduced, and in HCC patients

Liver diseases	**Alteration in gut microbiota**	**Clinical significance**	**References**
Chronic hepatitis C	*Streptococcus*↑ *Lactobacillus*↑ *Lachnospiraceae*↓ *Ruminococcaceae*↓	HCV infection cause gut microbial dysbiosis, even in mild liver patients	[31]
Chronic hepatitis B	*Actinomyces*↑ *Enterococcus faecalis*↑ *Alistipes*↓ *Bifidobacteria*↓	Gut microbial dysbiosis may effect disease development	[32]
ALD	*Lachnospiraceae*↑ *Erysipelotrichaceae*↑ *Lactobacillus*↓ *Pediococcus*↓	ALD induced by alcohol and stimulate bacterial disruption in microbial dysbiosis	[33]
NASH (fibrosis)	*Escherichia Shigella*↑ *Bacteroides*↑ *Clostridium*↓ *Prevotella*↓	These pathogens are primary contributor to NAFLD development	[34]
NAFLD	*Escherichia_Shigella*↑ *Blautia*↑ *Prevotellaceae*↓ *Ruminococcaceae*↓	The decreased pathogens are detrimental for adults with NAFLD	[34]
Liver cirrhosis	*Enterobacteriaceae* ↑ *Streptococcaceae*↑ *Lachnospiraceae* ↓ *Bacteroidaceae* ↓	Liver cirrhosis development linked with gut microbial dysbiosis	[35]
HCC patients	Lipopolysaccharide producing bacteria↑ *Escherichia coli*↑ Butyrate-producing bacteria↓	Cirrhotic patients with are more susceptible to the to HCC progression by stimulating tumor growth	[36]

Table 2.
Alteration in gut microbiota in various liver diseases.

DOI: http://dx.doi.org/10.5772/intechopen.106020

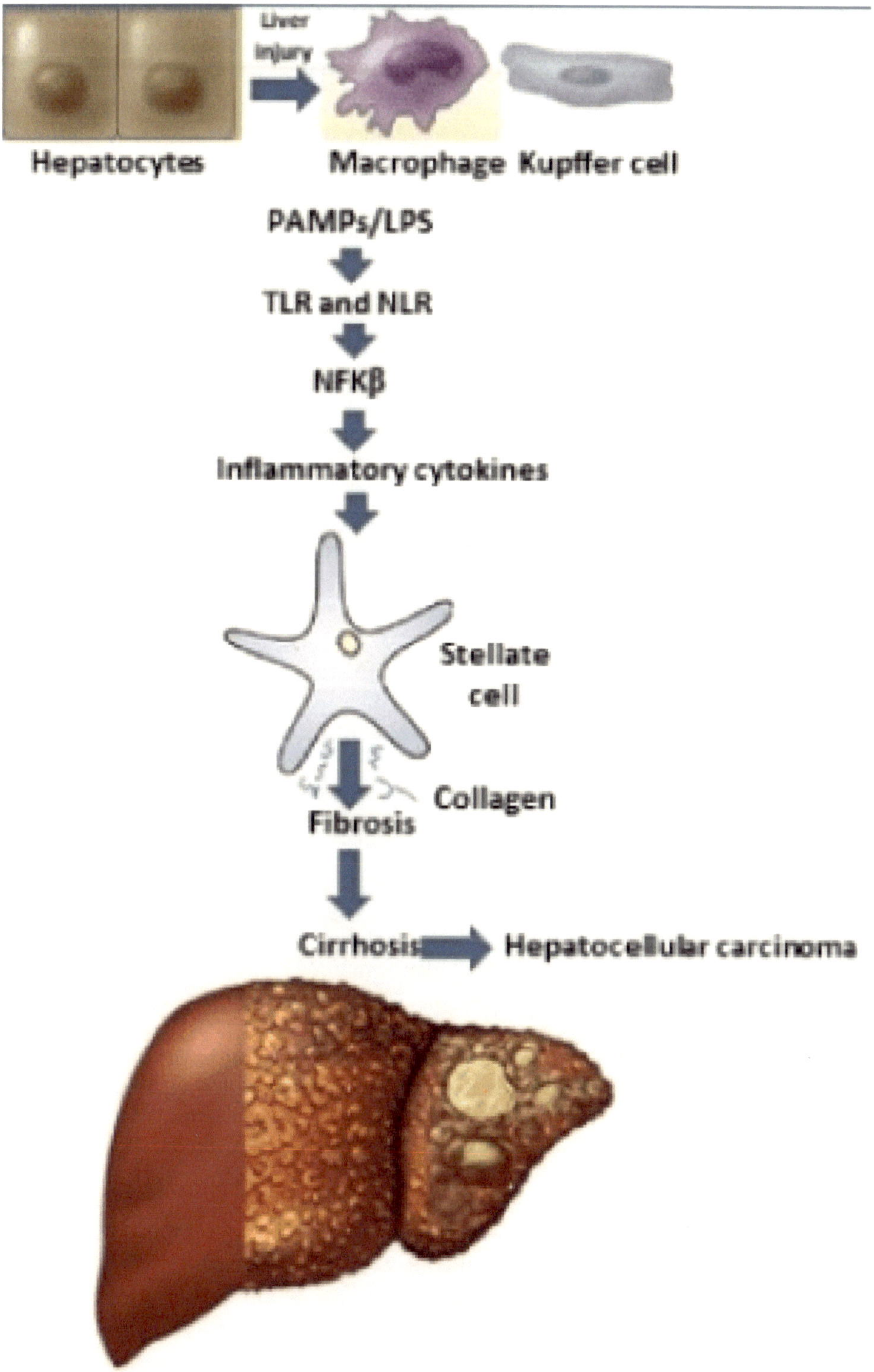

Figure 3.
Activation of immune system in HCC [15].

the levels of Escherichia coli and other gram-negative bacteria upsurge in as described in **Table 2**. Moreover, along with microbial alteration energy-producing system, microbial metabolism and iron transport also differ in hepatic carcinoma patients and healthy people. The levels of and serum tumor necrosis factor (TNF-α), LSM levels, fecal secretory IgA and gene diversity index significantly increased, and these features of gut microbial dysbiosis affect disease progression [37, 38].

The relationship of gut microbial dysbiosis and HCC is complex. The pathogenic micro-organisms antigen pass through the gut epithelium and recognized by dendritic cells, which stimulate the adaptive immune system by altering the T cells response to influence the development of HCC. For instance, T helper 17 (Th17) cells are a unique subcategory of T helper cells, to produce inflammatory cytokines and angiogenic mediators such as IL-17A and IL-22. IL-17A, that eventually activate tumor angiogenesis. Moreover, pathogen-associated molecular patterns (PAMPs), including LPS, peptidoglycans, and flagelin stimulate NFKβ with the help of toll-like receptors (TLRs) and nod-like receptors (NLRs), which also leads to produce inflammatory chemokines and cytokines, which enter the liver by portal circulation. However, Kupffer cells are affect the LPS as compared to hepatocytes, while PAMPs activate stellate cells, which promote and progress fibrosis and HCC (**Figure 3**) [37].

4. Current therapies and their limitations

The several therapeutic approaches to treat HCC focus on the alteration of the processes such as cell cycle, apoptosis, and signal pathways. The treatments are classified into different categories which are described as follows.

4.1 Pharmacological therapy

Sorafenib is the manifold kinase inhibitor, which suppresses the activity of Raf-1 and some other tyrosine kinases, like vascular VEGFR-2, VEGFR-3, PDGFR, and FGFR-1 involved in cellular angiogenesis, proliferation, differentiation and survival. It is the front-line therapy and as first drug approved for systemic treatment of advanced HCC patients, who moderately conserved liver functions and not considered suitable for surgical resection or liver transplantation. The evidence showed that sorafenib response is mainly linked with correction of irregular glycosylation in erythroblastosis 26–1 (Ets-1) protein in HCC cells by promoting survival rate significantly, only in advanced HCC patients. A lot of patients quickly develop resistance against sorafenib. Therefore, Lenvatinib is an effective drug for the those HCC patients, in which surgery is not effective and they are resistant to sorafenib, but their survival rate can be increased by decreeing lymphangiogenesis and angiogenesis responses. Regorafenib is also a second-line oral drug which was developed by Bayer and it was FDA-approved in June 2017 for unresectable HCC. Ramuciruma is a drug which inhibit the binding of the VEGFR ligands as a human anti-VEGFR-2 monoclonal antibody. Drug resistant is always an issue for numerous drugs and their adverse side effects, such as sorafenib and lenvatinib cause hypertension, diarrhea and decreased appetite [15, 39].

4.2 Surgery

Surgery of HCC patients includes three main categories such as surgical resection, adjuvant therapy after surgical resection and liver transplantation. Surgical resection is the HCC treatment for those patients who preserved liver function. The advancement of laparoscopic liver resection declines the operative blood loss, operation time, and length of hospital stay. If the surgical resection is done in early HCC (5 cm) patients with maximum preserved liver function, then the 5-yr survival rate can be 40–70%. The drawback of surgical resection is recurrence and its possible treatments include repeat hepatectomy, radiofrequency ablation, or salvage liver transplantation. After surgical resection, adjuvant therapy eliminates remaining cancer cells and inhibit secondary liver carcinogenesis. These therapies comprise of intra-arterial radiolabeled lip iodol, interferons, systemic and intra-arterial chemotherapy, acyclic retinoid, adoptive immunotherapy and sorafenib. The liver transplantation decreases postoperative liver failure risk, and best approach for moderate to severe cirrhosis or early-stage HCC patients. The liver transplant increase survival rate at 10 years which is more than liver resection, but the risks are there because of unacceptability of the donor liver by the body and cause high expense of short-term mortality [3, 40].

4.3 Loco-regional therapy

Loco-regional ablative therapy includes cryotherapy, ethanol injection and radiofrequency ablation. This therapy is the primary treatment for those HCC patients who are not capable of operation and it act as a bridge to liver transplantation or relaxing process to prolong the disease-free survival. For instance, radiofrequency ablation (RFA) is the process of coagulative necrosis for the thermal destruction of HCC cells and it is considered as far better than percutaneous ethanol injection (PEI), which is ablative therapy for early HCC patients. Moreover, RFA highly reduce the risk of morbidity in small HCC patients as compared to liver resection [41].

4.4 Cytotoxic chemotherapy

Chemotherapy is particularly workable for the patients with underlying non-cirrhotic liver. Chemotherapy cannot be used routinely for advanced HCC patients because HCC is chemotherapy-refractory tumor. Moreover, systemic chemotherapy is not tolerated by patients with underlying hepatic dysfunction. There are various chemotherapeutic agents, such as single-agent doxorubicin has an objective response rate of 20% or less with doses of 75 mg/m2 in advanced HCC patients. Systematic chemotherapy has limited efficacy on HCC because of low response rates and high toxicity, without increasing the significant survival rate such as gemcitabine- and doxorubicin-based chemotherapy treatment [3].

4.5 Natural compounds

Various natural compounds in fruits, vegetables, and spices function are helpful in suppressing mechanisms of cancer progression and in activating mechanisms of cancer prevention. These compounds promote anti-inflammatory, anti-oxidant, anti-tumor and anti-proliferative systems. Some compounds cause cytotoxicity to cancer cells and no effect on non-cancerous cells. For example, piperine is a natural compound, which inhibit enzymes of drug metabolism and it can be used in future as co-administrative with chemotherapeutic drugs to upsurge plasma concentrations. Some other natural compounds such as curcumin, oleocanthal, allium extracts and *Cnidium officinale* makino, also used to reduce HCC progression. The natural compounds may improve the effectiveness of current drug treatments without host toxicity. For instance, polysaccharides from *Lentinus edodes* and *Tricholoma matsutake* improve the inhibitory effect of 5-fluorouracil in H22 cells of HCC patients [42].

4.6 Oncolytic virus therapy

Oncolytic virus therapy is a new anticancer approach which involve replication of oncolytic viruses in carcinogenic tissues to lyse tumor cells. They are specially designed agents such as antitumor, tumor-selective and multi-mechanistic such as extending from direct killing of virus-mediated cancer cells, pleiotropic cytotoxic immune effector process, by the exact transgene-encoded proteins activities. The viruses of different classes used in this process such as paramyxovirus, reovirus, herpes, simplex virus, parvovirus, poxvirus and adenovirus. Some of these viruses are genetically engineered to improve their therapeutic effects. The oncolytic viruses also activate immunogenic tumor cell death and regulate cellular tumor– resistance mechanisms which leads to identification of recently released tumor antigens by producing tumor cell lysates. Moreover, in HCC oncolytic viruses such as telomerase-specific replication, telomelysin (OBP-301) and competent oncolytic adenovirus established efficient replication in telomerase-positive tumor cells, by replacing the adenoviral E1A promoter with the tumor-specific telomerase reverse transcriptase (hTERT) promoter [43].

4.7 Immunotherapy

The immune therapeutic approaches in HCC, target tumor cells by activation and stimulation of the current tumor-specific immune response. In this therapy, the patients are treated with advanced melanoma by immune-checkpoint-mechanism inhibitors including anti –cytotoxic T-lymphocyte antigen 4 (CTLA-4) antibody. The programmed death 1 (PD-1), is a co-inhibitory receptor, which is dominated by activated T and B cells, and regulate peripheral immune tolerance. Furthermore, the in PD-1 and its ligands interactions such as programmed death ligand 1 (PD-L1) (B7-H1) and PD-L2 (B7-DC), is an immune suppressant mechanism and a vital immune barrier. Other immunotherapies include tumor-associated antigens (TAAs) recognition by cytotoxic T lymphocytes (CTLs) to improve host immunity. The HCC tumor has TAA, cyclophilin B, as a squamous cell cancerous antigen recognized by T cells (SART) 2, SART3, AFP, hTERT, glycopican-3 (GPC3), and melanoma antigen gene A (MAGE-A). The drug sorafenib inhibit immunosuppression, therefore can be considered as immunotherapy combination with this drug [41].

4.8 Nanotechnology

Nanotechnology is an emerging technique which modify the concept of current combination therapy methods and increase retention, permeability and pharmacokinetics. The nanoparticles approach is treatment programs which syndicate the separate agents to increase the effects of drug. For instance, in combination as chemosensitize cancer cells become resistant to drugs and to improve the drug's efficacy in treating tumors, nanoparticles improve the results by the addition of another molecule in the mechanism. In HepG2 cells, doxorubicin delivery and the lipid nanoparticle as chemo-sensitizer release over 48 h and led to possible synergy, to a decrease in cytotoxicity than free doxorubicin and doxorubicin-nanoparticles. In case of diethylnitrosamine-causing liver cancers, doxorubicin/curcumin approach than free doxorubicin/curcumin act as a synergistic inhibition of tumors growth [42, 44].

5. Conclusion

Liver cancer comprises of different types depend upon their origin such as liver stem cells, hepatocytes, cholangiocytes, and hepatoblasts, the most common type is hepatocellular carcinoma (HCC) or primary liver cancer Worldwide, its prevalence is 75% of all types of liver cancers and every fifth male and seventh in female is diagnosed with liver cancer. The etiology is linked with activation of multiple processes of apoptotic response, dysregulation of cell cycle and the stimulation of signaling pathways that cause fibrogenic and inflammatory response. Currently, numerous therapeutic options are working to treat patients with HCC, the aim of all of these approaches is to improve liver function, overall survival, and life quality of patients, but only a few of these bioactive techniques have shown successful responses without initiating side effects.

6. Future perspective

Although, various drugs have been tested and approved for advanced HCC, but one of the main reasons of low survival rate is drug resistance because of the intratumor heterogeneity during treatment. This is a huge hurdle for the long-term use of targeted therapies for primary liver cancer, that is why it is essential to explore the mechanism of drug resistance in future. Another challenge for targeted treatments is the deficiency of accurate targets and biomarkers such as breast cancer has the exact biomarker like HER2, but primary liver cancer has no accurate biomarkers and show heterogeneity and genomic diversity. While many mutant genes such as TERT and CTNNB1, have been found, but it is still not clear as they are driver gene or passenger gene in future, it is essential to understand the genomic architecture, mutation landscape, and driver genes to use new therapeutic interventions. Most of the patients are not adaptable to immune therapy, therefore future efforts in should be made in two directions for immunotherapy such as improving the existing immune response and stimulating a new immune response. Moreover, further study is undoubtedly compulsory to advance improvement in current diagnosis, to better comprehend the genomic profile and pathogenesis of HCC to develop novel therapeutics, containing multiple drugs or treatments, that capable of modifying various signaling and biological pathways associated with HCC pathogenesis.

Author details

Aqsa Nazir[1*], Muhammad Aqib[2] and Muhammad Usman[2]

1 Institute of Food Science and Technology, University of Agriculture Faisalabad, Pakistan

2 Department Nutritional Sciences, Government College University, Faisalabad, Pakistan

*Address all correspondence to: maqibniaz595@gmail.com

References

[1] Wang G, Wang Q, Liang N, Xue H, Yang T, Chen X, et al. Oncogenic driver genes and tumor microenvironment determine the type of liver cancer. Cell Death & Disease. 2020;**11**(5):1-13

[2] World Health Organization. Projections of Mortality and Causes of Death, 2016 to 2060. Geneva, Switzerland: World Health Organization; 2020 Available from: http://www.who.int/healthinfo/global_burden_disease/projections/en/

[3] Liu C-Y, Chen K-F, Chen P-J. Treatment of liver cancer. Cold Spring Harbor Perspectives in Medicine. 2015;**5**(9):a021535

[4] Singal AG, El-Serag HB. Hepatocellular carcinoma from epidemiology to prevention: Translating knowledge into practice. Clinical Gastroenterology and Hepatology. 2015;**13**(12):2140-2151

[5] Petrick JL, McGlynn KA. The changing epidemiology of primary liver cancer. Current epidemiology reports. 2019;**6**(2):104-111

[6] Petrick JL, Campbell PT, Koshiol J, Thistle JE, Andreotti G, Beane-Freeman LE, et al. Tobacco, alcohol use and risk of hepatocellular carcinoma and intrahepatic cholangiocarcinoma: The liver cancer pooling project. British Journal of Cancer. 2018;**118**(7):1005-1012

[7] Lushniak BD, Samet JM, Pechacek TF, Norman LA, Taylor PA. The Health Consequences of Smoking—50 Years of Progress: A Report of the Surgeon General. Atlanta, GA, USA: Centers for disease control and Prevention; 2014

[8] Groopman JD, Smith JW, Rivera-Andrade A, Alvarez CS, Kroker-Lobos MF, Egner PA, et al. Aflatoxin and the aetiology of liver cancer and its implications for Guatemala. World Mycotoxin Journal. 2021;**14**(3):305-317

[9] Ogunwobi OO, Harricharran T, Huaman J, Galuza A, Odumuwagun O, Tan Y, et al. Mechanisms of hepatocellular carcinoma progression. World Journal of Gastroenterology. 2019;**25**(19):2279

[10] Tansel A, Katz LH, El-Serag HB, Thrift AP, Parepally M, Shakhatreh MH, et al. Incidence and determinants of hepatocellular carcinoma in autoimmune hepatitis: A systematic review and meta-analysis. Clinical Gastroenterology and Hepatology. 2017;**15**(8):1207-1217

[11] Marquardt JU, Andersen JB, Thorgeirsson SS. Functional and genetic deconstruction of the cellular origin in liver cancer. Nature Reviews Cancer. 2015;**15**(11):653-667

[12] Refolo MG, Messa C, Guerra V, Carr BI, D'alessandro R. Inflammatory mechanisms of HCC development. Cancers. 2020;**12**(3):641

[13] Yang YM, Kim SY, Seki E. Inflammation and liver cancer: Molecular mechanisms and therapeutic targets. In: Seminars in Liver Disease. Vol. 39, No. 1. New York, NY, USA: Thieme Medical Publishers; 2019. pp. 26-42

[14] Marquardt JU, Seo D, Andersen JB, Gillen MC, Kim MS, Conner EA, et al. Sequential transcriptome analysis of human liver cancer indicates late stage acquisition of malignant traits. Journal of Hepatology. 2014;**60**(2):346-353

[15] Galicia-Moreno M, Silva-Gomez JA, Lucano-Landeros S, Santos A, Monroy-Ramirez HC, Armendariz-Borunda J. Liver cancer: Therapeutic challenges and the importance of experimental models. Canadian Journal of Gastroenterology and Hepatology. 2021;**2021**:8837811

[16] Guo L, Teng L. YAP/TAZ for cancer therapy: Opportunities and challenges. International Journal of Oncology. 2015;**46**(4):1444-1452

[17] Khalaf AM, Fuentes D, Morshid AI, Burke MR, Kaseb AO, Hassan M, et al. Role of Wnt/β-catenin signaling in hepatocellular carcinoma, pathogenesis, and clinical significance. Journal of hepatocellular carcinoma. 2018;**5**:61

[18] Czauderna C, Castven D, Mahn FL, Marquardt JU. Context-dependent role of NF-κB signaling in primary liver cancer—From tumor development to therapeutic implications. Cancers. 2019;**11**(8):1053

[19] McVicker BL, Hamel FG, Simpson RL, Bennett RG. A selective PPARγ modulator reduces hepatic fibrosis. Biology. 2020;**9**(7):151

[20] Dong Y, Wang A. Aberrant DNA methylation in hepatocellular carcinoma tumor suppression. Oncology Letters. 2014;**8**(3):963-968

[21] Heo MJ, Yun J, Kim SG. Role of non-coding RNAs in liver disease progression to hepatocellular carcinoma. Archives of Pharmacal Research. 2019;**42**(1):48-62

[22] Liu Y-X, Li Q-Z, Cao Y-N, Zhang L-Q. Identification of key genes and important histone modifications in hepatocellular carcinoma. Computational and Structural Biotechnology Journal. 2020;**18**:2657-2669

[23] Svinka J, Mikulits W, Eferl R. STAT3 in hepatocellular carcinoma: New perspectives. Hepatic Oncology. 2014;**1**(1):107-120

[24] Wang N, Wang S, Li M-Y, Hu B-g, Liu L-p, Yang S-l, et al. Cancer stem cells in hepatocellular carcinoma: An overview and promising therapeutic strategies. Therapeutic Advances in Medical Oncology. 2018;**10**:1-25

[25] Yin F, Han X, Yao S-K, Wang X-L, Yang H-C. Importance of SALL4 in the development and prognosis of hepatocellular carcinoma. World Journal of Gastroenterology. 2016;**22**(9):2837

[26] Guichard C, Amaddeo G, Imbeaud S, Ladeiro Y, Pelletier L, Maad IB, et al. Integrated analysis of somatic mutations and focal copy-number changes identifies key genes and pathways in hepatocellular carcinoma. Nature Genetics. 2012;**44**(6):694-698

[27] Zhang N, Bai H, David KK, Dong J, Zheng Y, Cai J, et al. The Merlin/NF2 tumor suppressor functions through the YAP oncoprotein to regulate tissue homeostasis in mammals. Developmental Cell. 2010;**19**(1):27-38

[28] Lanaya H, Natarajan A, Komposch K, Li L, Amberg N, Chen L, et al. EGFR has a tumour-promoting role in liver macrophages during hepatocellular carcinoma formation. Nature Cell Biology. 2014;**16**(10):972-981

[29] Marquardt JU, Gomez-Quiroz L, Arreguin LO, Camacho FP, Lee Y-H, Kitade M, et al. Curcumin effectively inhibits oncogenic NF-κB signaling and restrains stemness features in liver cancer. Journal of Hepatology. 2015;**63**(3):661-669

[30] Jiang J-W, Chen X-H, Ren Z, Zheng S-S. Gut microbial dysbiosis associates

hepatocellular carcinoma via the gut-liver axis. Hepatobiliary & Pancreatic Diseases International. 2019;**18**(1): 19-27

[31] Inoue T, Nakayama J, Moriya K, Kawaratani H, Momoda R, Ito K, et al. Gut dysbiosis associated with hepatitis C virus infection. Clinical Infectious Diseases. 2018;**67**(6):869-877

[32] Wang J, Yang Wang X, Zhang JL, Qianpeng Zhang Y, Zhao JP, et al., editors. Gut microbial dysbiosis is associated with altered hepatic functions and serum metabolites in chronic hepatitis B patients. Frontiers in Microbiology. 2017;**8**:2222

[33] Yan AW, Fouts DE, Brandl J, Stärkel P, Torralba M, Schott E, et al. Enteric dysbiosis associated with a mouse model of alcoholic liver disease. Hepatology. 2011;**53**(1):96-105

[34] Shen F, Zheng R-D, Sun X-Q, Ding W-J, Wang X-Y, Fan J-G. Gut microbiota dysbiosis in patients with non-alcoholic fatty liver disease. Hepatobiliary & Pancreatic Diseases International. 2017;**16**(4):375-381

[35] Qin N, Yang F, Li A, Prifti E, Chen Y, Shao L, et al. Alterations of the human gut microbiome in liver cirrhosis. Nature. 2014;**513**(7516):59-64

[36] Ren Z, Li A, Jiang J, Lin Z, Yu Z, Lu H, et al. Gut microbiome analysis as a tool towards targeted non-invasive biomarkers for early hepatocellular carcinoma. Gut. 2019;**68**(6):1014-1023

[37] Milosevic I, Vujovic A, Barac A, Djelic M, Korac M, Spurnic AR, et al. Gut-liver axis, gut microbiota, and its modulation in the management of liver diseases: A review of the literature. International Journal of Molecular Sciences. 2019;**20**(2):395

[38] Zhou A, Tang L, Zeng S, Lei Y, Yang S, Tang B. Gut microbiota: A new piece in understanding hepatocarcinogenesis. Cancer Letters. 2020;**474**:15-22

[39] Jindal A, Thadi A, Shailubhai K. Hepatocellular carcinoma: Etiology and current and future drugs. Journal of Clinical and Experimental Hepatology. 2019;**9**(2):221-232

[40] Kamiyama T, Tahara M, Nakanishi K, Yokoo H, Kamachi H, Kakisaka T, et al. Long-term outcome of laparoscopic hepatectomy in patients with hepatocellular carcinoma. Hepato-Gastroenterology. 2014;**61**(130):405-409

[41] Feng Q, Chi Y, Liu Y, Zhang L, Liu Q. Efficacy and safety of percutaneous radiofrequency ablation versus surgical resection for small hepatocellular carcinoma: A meta-analysis of 23 studies. Journal of Cancer Research and Clinical Oncology. 2015;**141**(1):1-9

[42] Anwanwan D, Singh SK, Singh S, Saikam V, Singh R. Challenges in liver cancer and possible treatment approaches. Biochimica et Biophysica Acta (BBA)-Reviews on Cancer. 2020;**1873**(1):188314

[43] Russell SJ, Peng K-W, Bell JC. Oncolytic virotherapy. Nature Biotechnology. 2012;**30**(7):658-670

[44] Ballout F, Habli Z, Rahal ON, Fatfat M, Gali-Muhtasib H. Thymoquinone-based nanotechnology for cancer therapy: Promises and challenges. Drug Discovery Today. 2018;**23**(5):1089-1098

Chapter 2

Non-alcoholic Fatty Liver Disease Associated Hepatocellular Carcinoma

Kai Sun, Alan Hodges and Maen Abdelrahim

Abstract

Non-alcoholic fatty liver disease (NAFLD) is a spectrum of diseases ranging from non-alcoholic fatty liver and non-alcoholic steatohepatitis to its more severe forms such as liver fibrosis and cirrhosis. The incidence of hepatocellular carcinoma (HCC) increases as NAFLD progresses to the more severe forms. As prevalence of obesity and metabolic syndrome rising in North America, NAFLD associated HCC is becoming the leading cause of HCC. Different from other causes of HCC, altered metabolic state and its impact on immune response play an important role in the pathogenesis of NAFLD associated HCC. Currently, immune checkpoint inhibitors and combination therapy are first-line treatments of advanced HCC regardless of etiologies. Given the rising incidence of NAFLD associated HCC and its unique pathogenesis, future clinical trials should assess whether HCC etiology—NAFLD in particular—influence the safety and efficacy of a given treatment.

Keywords: hepatocellular carcinoma, non-alcoholic fatty liver disease, non-alcoholic steatohepatitis, liver cirrhosis, tyrosine kinase inhibitor, immunotherapy

1. Introduction

Non-alcoholic fatty liver disease (NAFLD) is defined as the presence of >= 5% hepatic fat accumulation of the liver in the absence of other causes of fatty liver disease. NAFLD is a spectrum of diseases. In its mildest form- non-alcoholic fatty liver (NAFL, also known as simple hepatic steatosis)- fat accumulation is seen in the liver but without significant inflammation or hepatocellular injury. The next stage of NAFLD is non-alcoholic steatohepatitis (NASH) which is characterized by histological lobular inflammation and hepatocyte ballooning. The condition then progresses to liver fibrosis and accumulation of fibrosis leads to liver cirrhosis [1]. In studies [2–5] that examined paired liver biopsies in patients with baseline NAFLD, up to 20–40% patients with NAFL can progress to fibrosis over an average follow-up between 2.2 and 13.8 years. In a meta-analysis including 411 patients with NAFLD, 35.8%, 32.5%, 16.7%, 9.3%, and 5.7% patients exhibited stage 0,1,2,3,4 fibrosis, respectively with an average fibrosis progression of 0.07 stages per year [6]. The rate of progression is twice as high in patients with NASH and a subgroup of both NASH and NAFL patients may rapidly progress from no fibrosis to advanced fibrosis over an average of six years [3, 7].

NAFLD is considered the hepatic manifestation of metabolic syndrome and many other manifestations of metabolic syndrome including obesity and type 2 diabetes mellitus (T2DM) are independent risk factors of NAFLD. As metabolic syndrome becomes epidemic, the predicted prevalence of obesity will reach close to 50% by year 2030 [8], and the projected NAFLD prevalence among the adult population (aged ≥15 years) will rise to 33.5% [9]. NAFLD-associated hepatocellular carcinoma (HCC) cases are expected to increase by 146% from 10,100 to 24,900 during 2015–2030 and become the leading cause of HCC.

This chapter summaries the current knowledge on the diagnosis, epidemiology, pathogenesis, and treatment of NAFLD associated HCC. It highlights the unique pathogenesis of NALFD associated HCC and discusses challenges we face with current treatment.

2. Definition and diagnosis of NAFLD

Liver biopsy remains the gold standard of diagnosing NAFL, NASH, liver fibrosis and cirrhosis. However, due to its invasive nature, imaging modalities are commonly utilized for diagnosing different stages of NAFLD. Ultrasound and computed tomography (CT) are the most commonly used fist-line investigation with generally good sensitivity and specificity [10–12]. However, the sensitivity lowers when the level of steatosis is low [13]. Other techniques such as transient elastography MRI, MRI elastography, computer-assisted quantitative techniques have been developed to better assess steatosis and fibrosis [14–17]. These techniques are not widely available and could associate with high cost. Simple biochemical markers such as low albumin, prolonged prothrombin time and thrombocytopenia should be incorporated into the diagnostic algorithm of NAFLD as well [1]. If a diagnosis is uncertain with imaging modalities or if there a high probability of liver fibrosis, a liver biopsy is warranted.

3. Epidemiology of NAFLD-associated HCC

3.1 Incidence of NAFLD-associated HCC

NAFLD is the fastest growing cause of HCC in the world. As only a small proportion of patients undergo screening and appropriate surveillance [18], it is extremely difficult to get representative estimates of HCC incidence in the general population with NAFLD. Thus, studies are limited to patients who underwent appropriate workup and surveillance. Given that diagnoses of the exact NAFLD stage can be challenging, the percentage of patients with NAFL, NASH and cirrhosis is unclear without definitive liver biopsy in most published studies. In one large population based study, the incidence of HCC in patients with NAFLD is estimated at 0.51% at year 12 [19]. The incidence of HCC increases as NAFLD progresses from NAFL to cirrhosis with the highest HCC incidence rate seen in those with NAFLD-associated liver cirrhosis. HCC incidence in patients with NAFL is low at 1.2 per 1000 person-years in a population-based study of US Veterans [20] and ranges from 0.3% to 0.43% in other studies that excluded patients with cirrhosis [19, 21, 22]. In contrast, HCC incidence in patients with cirrhosis dramatically rises to about 10 per 1000 person-years in the same US Veterans study [20], and could be up to 12.8% over 3 years in a systemic review [22].

NAFLD-associated HCC is becoming the leading cause of HCC as the prevalence of obesity and metabolic syndrome is rising. The increasing prevalence of NAFLD-associated HCC is reflected in studies utilizing large national transplant registries. Based on the data from the Scientific Registry of Transplant Recipients (SRTR) data system from 2002 to 2017 [23], 17% patients who were listed for liver transplant had a listing diagnosis of HCC. Even though chronic hepatitis C remained the leading cause of HCC in these transplant candidates and had a 6.2-fold increase from 2002 to 2017, NAFLD-associated HCC had an 11.5-fold increase. NAFLD-associated HCC is the most rapidly growing indication for liver transplantation. It comprised of 18% of liver transplant candidates with HCC in 2017 in contrast with that of 2% in 2002, while chronic hepatitis C related HCC decreased to 48% in 2017 from 53% in 2002. According to a predictive model, NAFLD prevalence among the adult population (aged ≥15 years) is projected at 33.5% in 2030; among the NAFLD cases, NASH cases are expected to increase from 20% to 27% by 2030; incidence of decompensated cirrhosis will increase 168% to 105,430 cases by 2030; prevalent HCC cases are expected to increase by 146% from 10,100 to 24,900 during 2015–2030; incident HCC cases are expected to increase by 137% from 5,160 to 12,240 in 2030 [9]. With more curative treatments being developed for chronic hepatitis C, the incidence of chronic hepatitis C related HCC is expected to decrease, while NAFLD-associated HCC is becoming the leading cause of HCC.

3.2 Risk factors of NAFLD-associated HCC

Many of the NAFLD risk factors including obesity, metabolic syndrome and T2DM are also independent risk factors of HCC. Other demographic risk factors including older age, male sex, Hispanic ethnicity, and genetic predisposition have also been studied as risk factors in HCC, including NAFLD-associated HCC.

3.2.1 Obesity, T2DM and metabolic syndrome

Obesity is closely related to both NAFLD and HCC. Obesity is the most common metabolic abnormality associated with NAFLD: an estimated 51.3% patients with NAFLD had obesity and up to 81.8% patients with NASH were obese [24]. Obesity is associated with many types of malignancies including HCC. It is assumed that 10% or more liver cancers could be attributable to excess weight [25]. T2DM is found in up to 71% of patients with NASH cirrhosis and is independently associated with increased risk of HCC [26]. A Surveillance, Epidemiology, and End Results (SEER)-Medicare based study from 1993 to 2005 showed that up to 37.1% patients with HCC had metabolic syndrome in contrast with 17.1% of comparison group residing in the same regions as the SEER registries. Among the metabolic conditions, T2DM or impaired fasting glucose has the strongest association with HCC. Metabolic syndrome remained significantly associated with increased risk of HCC even after adjusted multiple logistic regression analyses, suggesting metabolic syndrome as an independent risk factor for developing HCC [27].

3.2.2 Demographic and genetic risk factors

NAFLD-associated HCC present at a later age and is more prevalent in male. Significant racial and ethnic disparities in NAFLD and NAFLD-associated HCC in the United States are seen. Hispanics have the highest risk of developing NAFLD and

NAFLD-associated HCC [28, 29]. Carriage of the PNPLA3 rs738409 C >G polymorphism is not only associated with greater risk of progressive steatohepatitis and fibrosis, but also of HCC with a 2.26-fold increased risk of HCC when carrying one copy of the allele, and 5-fold increased risk in homozygous individuals [30].

4. Pathogenesis of NAFLD associated HCC

NAFLD associated HCC is similar to many chronic liver disease related hepatocellular carcinomas, where hepatocellular injury and subsequent necroinflammation drive the formation of a protumorigenic microenvironment in the liver [31–33]. This microenvironment consists of a complex chronic inflammatory state with increased metabolic, oxidative, and mutagenic cellular stress, ultimately driving hepatocarcinogenesis (**Figure 1**) [31, 34, 35]. Different from other causes of HCC, e.g., viral or alcohol, an altered metabolomic state is the driver of hepatocellular injury in NAFLD associated HCC, playing an important role throughout the pathogenic process, and culminating in unique alterations of the molecular phenotype of the resulting tumor. The precise pathogenic mechanisms of NAFLD associated HCC continue to evolve, as the complex interplay of environmental factors, genetic susceptibility, and intricate inflammatory conditions further unfold.

4.1 Hepatocellular injury and the production of a protumorigenic microenvironment

The original model of hepatocellular injury in NASH was described as a "two-hit" hypothesis, where the first hit, steatosis, sensitizes the hepatocyte to injury and cell death resulting from the "second-hit" of oxidative stress [36]. Although this model is largely seen as overly reductive, it does provide a conceptual framework for hepatocellular injury in NAFLD associated HCC. Lipotoxicity, a state of lipid dysregulation

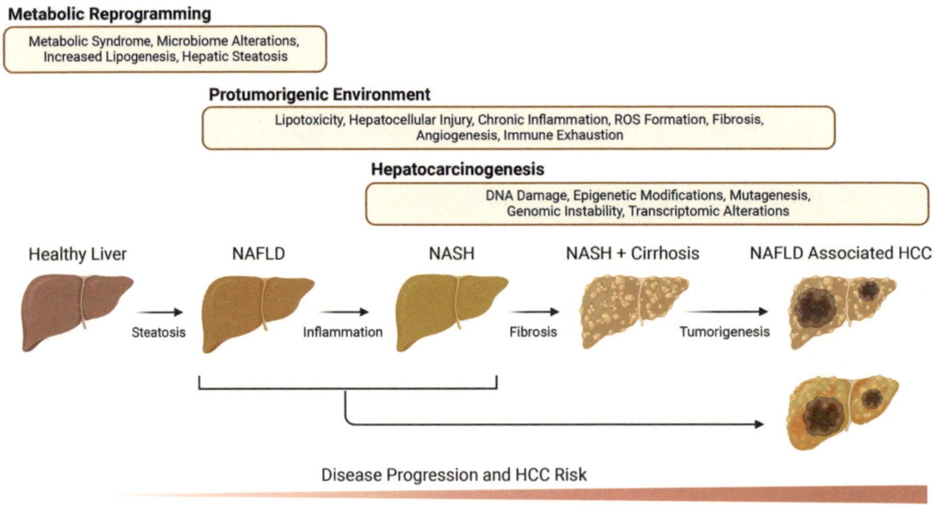

Figure 1.
Stepwise pathogenesis of NAFLD associated HCC. In the setting of environmental and genetic predisposition, the sequalae of metabolic reprograming and hepatocellular injury in NAFLD lead to the creation of a protumorigenic microenvironment and ultimately hepatocarcinogenesis. Created with BioRender.com.

leading to organelle dysfunction and cell death, is often-considered the initial metabolic insult that causes hepatocellular injury in NAFLD [32]. Increased hepatic lipid deposits are a hallmark of NAFLD. Multiple features of metabolic syndrome, including excess dietary free fatty acids (FFAs), excess FFA release from adipose tissue, increased insulin resistance, upregulated de-novo lipogenesis and alterations of the gut microbiota all contribute to a lipid-rich hepatic metabolic state [37]. At increased concentrations in the liver, lipids are directly and indirectly hepatotoxic, promoting proapoptotic and ER-stress pathways, while inducing mitochondrial dysfunction and reactive oxygen species (ROS) production [38]. In addition to lipid induced hepatocellular injury, derangements in other metabolic pathways seen in NAFLD, including bile acid metabolism and iron storage, likely contribute to hepatocyte damage and hepatocarcinogenesis as well [39, 40].

As in many cancers, the innate and adaptive immune system play a Janus-faced role in tumor development: both promoting necroinflammation and therefore carcinogenesis, while also performing antitumor cell killing and immune surveillance [41]. Hepatocellular injury in NAFLD plays a central role in disrupting this balancing act, skewing the immune response to favor tumorigenesis. Hepatocyte death stimulates the immune response through exposure of immune cells to damage associated molecular patterns (DAMPS). Additionally, microbiome changes in NAFLD patients likely contribute to the inflammatory immune phenotype, with the increased "leakiness" gut leading to increased translocation of lipopolysaccharide (LPS) and other pathogen associated molecular patterns (PAMPS) into the portal circulation [42]. Both DAMPS and PAMPS act through Toll-like receptors (TLR) and other pattern recognition receptors to activate liver resident macrophages (Kupffer cells). Activated Kupffer cells (KCs) recruit and stimulate other innate and adaptive immune cell subsets which secrete proinflammatory factors including IL-1β, IL-2, IL-7, IL-12, IL-15, TNFα, and IFNγ, further promoting an immunostimulatory and cytotoxic environment. A major consequence of the immunostimulatory environment is the activation of non-parenchymal hepatic cells including hepatic stellate cells, which increase extracellular matrix deposition and fibrosis. Moreover, stimulated innate cells directly contribute to the abundance of ROS and therefore oxidative DNA damage in the liver due to increased respiratory burst activity [41]. Together these immunostimulatory processes perpetuate hepatic cell death, promote hepatic stellate cell mediated fibrosis, and contribute genotoxic metabolites to the microenvironment, all key drivers of hepatocarcinogenesis. In response to these chronic inflammatory conditions, many immune exhaustion responses are induced, including the expression of immunosuppressive factors (IL-10, TGFβ) and the immune checkpoint PD-L1. While this immunosuppressive response contributes to the reduction of detrimental inflammation, antitumor cytotoxic immune response is inhibited as well, contributing to tumor growth.

In addition to the directly cytotoxic and genotoxic mechanisms described above, the positive feedback loop of hepatocellular injury, necroinflammation and fibrosis indirectly promote tumor progression through induction of angiogenesis. In response to inflammatory stimuli, activated monocytes increase production of VEGF and MMP9, promoting tumor neovascularization, growth, and metastasis [43]. Notably even prior to HCC development, NAFLD patients exhibit increased serologic markers of angiogenesis and increased neovascularization in biopsy samples [44], further contributing to the confluence of protumorigenic factors ultimately leading to tumorigenesis in NAFLD.

The influence of metabolic syndrome can be observed in each of these protumorigenic mechanisms, hepatocellular injury, chronic inflammation, immune exhaustion, and increased neovascularization. Many features of metabolic syndrome including hyperlipidemia, hyperglyceridemia, and obesity directly contribute to steatosis and lipotoxic hepatocellular injury. Adipocytes directly produce multiple inflammatory cytokines (TNFα, IL-6) and proangiogenic factors (VEGF, FDGF), likely contributing to oncogenic chronic inflammation, immune exhaustion, and angiogenesis [45]. Mouse models of NAFLD induced HCC highlight the importance of metabolic syndrome in HCC pathogenesis. In mice with diet ± activity modifications designed to recapitulate conditions common metabolic syndrome, the vast majority (60–89%) of mice develop HCC [46], suggesting a potent role of metabolic syndrome in HCC development.

4.2 Hepatocarcinogenesis and disease progression

Ultimately the protumorigenic microenvironment results in DNA damage and subsequent mutagenesis. DNA oxidative damage is a major contributor to mutagenesis in NAFLD associated HCC. The DNA oxidative stress marker 8-hydroxy-2′-deoxyguanosine (8-OHdG) in NAFLD associated HCC is increased compared to that of healthy patient livers or tumors from patients with viral and alcohol associated HCC [47]. 8-OHdG is an independent risk factor for hepatocarcinogenesis and therefore highlights the role of oxidative damage in HCC pathogenesis. In addition to genotoxic alterations from DNA oxidative damage, oxidative damage can cause epigenetic changes, which may play a role in HCC carcinogenesis. Epigenetic inactivation of tumor suppressor genes consistent with oxidative DNA damage response have been observed in NAFLD induced HCC patients [48]. Furthermore, alterations in DNA repair pathways may also contribute to genomic instability. Upregulation of DNA-dependent protein kinase, a central member of the error prone DNA repair mechanism non-homologous end joining (NHEJ), has been observed in NAFLD associated HCC [49]. Together these mechanisms lead to an increased mutagenic state in NAFLD associated HCC.

Although a wide variety of mutations have been documented in NAFLD associated HCC, hotspot genes and mutational signatures have been described. In a cohort of 80 patients with NAFLD associated HCC, the most frequently mutated genes were the telomerase (TERT) promoter (56%); the gene encoding beta-catenin, CTNNB1 (28%); the tumor suppressor, TP53 (18%); and the activin receptor, ACVR2A (10%) [35]. Notably, TERT promotor, CTNNB1 and TP53 are mutated at similar rates in HCC patients en masse regardless of etiology; however, mutations in ACVR2A are more enriched in patients with NAFLD associated HCC compared with that in other etiologies [50]. Transcriptionally, the majority of NAFLD-associated HCC tumors demonstrated upregulation of either the WNT–TGFβ or WNT–β-catenin oncogenic signaling pathways, highlighting the importance of both non-canonical and canonical WNT signaling in NAFLD associated HCC carcinogenesis [35]. Moreover, other transcriptional signatures consistent with underlying pathogenic features of NAFLD associated HCC are enriched in these patients including bile acid metabolism, oxidative stress, and inflammation-related gene signatures. Together these genomic and transcriptomic alterations drive malignant transformation and disease progression.

5. Current treatment of NAFLD-associated HCC

Current HCC treatment recommendations incorporate Barcelona Clinic Liver Cancer (BCLC) stage, liver lesion number and size, liver function and patient performance status [51]. Treatment modalities for localized disease include hepatic resection, ablation, and liver transplant for single or small lesions; chemoembolization and stereotactic radiation for larger, multiple unresectable lesions. These locoregional treatments seem to be equally effective regardless of HCC etiology. A comprehensive review on different locoregional treatment modalities in NAFLD-associated HCC has been published recently [52]. This chapter will focus on systemic therapies, especially immune checkpoint inhibitors in NAFLD-associated HCC.

5.1 Tyrosine kinase inhibitor (TKI)

5.1.1 Sorafenib

The Phase III SHARP trial established the efficacy of sorafenib, a multikinase inhibitor, which prolonged the median survival and median time to radiographic progression for patients with locally advanced or metastatic HCC [53]. A similar Phase III trial that was conducted in Asian-Pacific region observed similar results [54]. In the SHARP study, 48% patients had viral hepatitis as an etiology of HCC and the percentage of NAFLD-associated HCC is unknown. The subsequent published subgroup analysis of SHARP study patients and combined analysis of SHARP study and Asian-Pacific study patients didn't include NAFLD-associated HCC as a subgroup either [55, 56]. A recent presented study of 5201 patients with HCC treated with sorafenib found that there is no overall survival or adverse event difference between NAFLD-associated HCC and other etiology related HCC. However, patients with NAFLD-associated HCC were significantly older and sorafenib was commenced at more advanced stages. There were only 3.6% patients with NAFLD-associated HCC in the study, limiting the ability of drawing definite conclusions [57].

5.1.2 Lenvatinib

Lenvatinib, another multikinase inhibitor, showed non-inferiority to sorafenib in the Phase III REFLECT study [58]. Similar to SHARP study, patients in REFLECT study was characterized as having viral etiologic HCC or alcohol related HCC. The percentage of NALFD-associated HCC is unknown. A recently published multi-center retrospective study from Japan included 530 HCC patients treated with Lenvatinib [59]. The study compared the survival of 103 patients with NAFLD-associated HCC with that of 427 patients with HCC from other etiologies and revealed that progression free survival was statistically better in patients with NAFLD-associated HCC (9.3 vs. 7.5 months, P = 0.012), and overall survival was numerically better even though not statistically significant (20.5 vs. 16.9 months, P = 0.057).

5.1.3 Other TKIs

Regorafenib was approved as a second-line treatment for advanced HCC after progressing on sorafenib based on the Phase III RESORCE study [60]. Ramucirumab was also approved for the same indication after showing overall survival and progression free survival benefit in patients with advanced HCC in REACH-2 study [61]. Multikinase inhibitor cabozantinib improved survival and PFS in patients who have failed one or two lines of treatment in the study CELESTIAL and cabozantinib was the first approved third-line treatment for advanced HCC [62]. In these three studies, subgroup analysis didn't show different response to these TKIs according to HCC etiology. In a retrospective study that included 23.5% NAFLD-associated HCC also showed similar responses to regorafenib regardless of HCC etiologies. However, there were less than 10% of NAFLD-associated HCC patients included in RESORCE, REACH-2 and CELESTIAL studies. And there were less than 25 patients in the retrospective study mentioned above. The small number of patients enrolled in the studies limit definitive conclusions.

5.2 Immune checkpoint inhibitors

Checkpoint inhibitor single agent was first studied in the second line settings. Both nivolumab and pembrolizumab showed improved response rate in the early phase clinical trials [63, 64]. Based on the results from these studies, FDA granted accelerated approval for advanced HCC. Pembrolizumab was further tested in the second line setting in KEYNOTE 240 study. However, the study didn't meet the primary endpoint of superior combined OS and PFS [65]. Similarly, Phase III CheckMate 459 study comparing nivolumab with sorafenib in the first line setting didn't show superiority of nivolumab [66]. Combing nivolumab and ipilimumab at different dose and schedule was explored and doublet regimen has shown improved response rate up to 30% in the second line setting [67]. Phase III HIMALAYA study added tremelimumab to durvalumab and compared this regimen with sorafenib. The combination treatment improved overall survival compared to sorafenib and the final results are eagerly anticipated [68].

As with studies of TKIs in HCC, most studies of immune checkpoint inhibitors stratified patients to groups of HBV related, HCV related and uninfected, and the percentage of NAFLD-associated HCC in the uninfected group is unknown. Nevertheless, subgroup analysis in most of these studies showed comparable efficacy of immune checkpoint inhibitors in uninfected and overall population (**Table 1**).

5.3 Immune checkpoint inhibitor and VGEF inhibitor

The combination of immune checkpoint inhibitor atezolizumab and VEGF inhibitor bevacizumab in patients with locally advanced or metastatic HCC in the first setting has shown superior OS and PFS compared to sorafenib in IMbrave150 trial [69]. The median OS was 19.2 months with atezolizumab plus bevacizumab and 13.4 months with sorafenib (hazard ratio 0.66; 95% CI 0.52–0.85; $p < 0.001$). The median PFS was 6.9 and 4.3 months in the respective treatment groups (HR 0.65; 95% CI 0.53–0.81; $p < 0.001$). The combination was approved by FDA as first line treatment for HCC in 2020 and is the preferred first line treatment over single agent immune checkpoint inhibitor or TKIs in eligible patients.

The percentage of NAFLD-associated HCC is unknown in this study but 30% of the patients had no viral infection. In the subgroup analysis, uninfected patients with HCC seemed to have derived less benefit from the combination treatment compared to patients with viral hepatitis (HR for death 1.05; 95% CI 0.68–1.63) [70]. A previous animal study has demonstrated the existence of a CD8+PD-1+ subset of protumorigenic cells in NASH that favor the development of HCC and hamper response

Study name/phase of study	Drug(s)	Etiology and patient numbers	Endpoint and results
Single agent			
CheckMate 040/ Phase I/II	Nivolumab	N = 262 HBV = 25.2% HCV = 22.9% Uninfected = 51.9%	ORR (CR+PR) 20% HBV 14% HCV 20% Uninfected 21–23%
CheckMate 459/ Phase III	Nivolumab vs. sorafenib	N = 743 (371 vs. 372) HBV = 31% HCV = 23% Uninfected = 45%	OS 16.4m vs. 14.7m ORR (CR+PR) 15% vs. 7% HBV 19% vs. 8% HCV 17% vs. 7% Uninfected 12% vs. 7%
Keynote 224/ Phase II	Pembrolizumab	N = 104 HBV 21% HCV 25% Uninfected 33%	ORR (CR+PR) 18.3% Infected (HBV+HCV) 13% Uninfected 20%
Keynote 240/Phase III	Pembrolizumab vs. BSC	N = 413 HBV 21.5–25.9% HCV 15.5–15.6% Uninfected 58.6–63.0%	OS and PFS* OS 13.9m vs. 10.6 m PFS 3.0m vs. 2.8 m
Doublet			
HIMALAYA/Phase III	Tremelimumab+durvalumab vs. sorafenib	N = 1171 HBV 30.6–31% HCV 27.5–28% Nonviral 41–41.9%	OS 16.43 m vs. 13.77 m
CheckMate 040/ Phase I/II	Nivolumab + ipilimumab#	N = 148 HBV 51% HCV 22% Uninfected 22%	ORR (CR+PR) ^ 27–32%

Abbreviations: HBV: hepatitis B; HCV: hepatitis C; BSC: best supportive care; ORR: objective response rate; CR: complete remission; PR: partial remission; OS: overall survival; PFS: progression free survival. *OS hazard ratios in patients with HBV, HCV and uninfected were 0.57 (0.35–0.94), 0.96 (0.48–1.92) and 0.88 (0.64–1.20) respectively. PFS hazard ratios in patients with HBV, HCV and uninfected were 0.70 (0.44–1.13), 0.46 (0.24–0.90), 0.75 (0.56–1.01).*

#Arm A: nivolumab 1 mg/kg plus ipilimumab 3 mg/kg, administered every 3 weeks (4 doses), followed by nivolumab 240 mg every 2 weeks; Arm B: nivolumab 3 mg/kg plus ipilimumab 1 mg/kg, administered every 3 weeks (4 doses), followed by nivolumab 240 mg every 2 weeks; Arm C: nivolumab 3 mg/kg every 2 weeks plus ipilimumab 1 mg/kg every 6 weeks (arm C).

^Median overall survival of patients who were HBV/HCV uninfected, HBV infected, or HCV infected in arm A was 22.2 months, 22.8 months, and 14.9 months; in arm B, 11.8 months, 12.1 months, and 16.1 months; and in arm C, 7.4 months, 9.6 months, and 33.0 months, respectively.

Table 1.
Overview of outcomes of checkpoint inhibitor studies in patients with locally advanced or metastatic hepatocellular carcinoma.

to immune checkpoint inhibitors. The authors also performed meta-analysis using data from CheckMate 459, IMbrave150 and KEYNOTE240, and revealed that patients with non-viral etiology had inferior survival when treated with immune checkpoint inhibitors. They then performed a cohort study of 130 patients with HCC from various etiologies and patients with NAFLD associated HCC had shorter overall survival of 5.4 months vs. 11 months in patients with HCC from other etiologies.

The better response to immunotherapy in patients with viral-induced HCC than in patients with NAFLD associated HCC might be due to the amount or quality of viral antigens or to a different liver micro-environment, possibly one that does not impair immune surveillance. Stratifying clinical trials according to HCC etiology for prospective validation in future clinical trials is warranted.

6. Conclusions

As incidence of HBV and HCV associated HCC continues to decrease with effective antiviral treatment, NAFLD associated HCC is becoming the leading cause of HCC. In light of the rising prevalence of NAFLD associated HCC, its unique pathogenesis and findings suggestive inferior response to immune checkpoint inhibitors, future clinical trials should assess whether HCC etiology influence the efficacy of a given treatment.

Conflict of interest

The authors declare no conflict of interest.

Author details

Kai Sun[1], Alan Hodges[2,3] and Maen Abdelrahim[1*]

1 Houston Methodist Neal Cancer Center, Houston, Texas, United States

2 Houston Methodist Research Institute, Center for Immunotherapy Research, Houston, Texas, United States

3 Texas A&M College of Medicine, Bryan, Texas, United States

*Address all correspondence to: mabdelrahim@houstonmethodist.org

References

[1] Jennison E, Patel J, Scorletti E, Byrne CD. Diagnosis and management of non-alcoholic fatty liver disease. Postgraduate Medical Journal. 2019;**95**(1124):314-322

[2] Wong VW, Wong GL, Choi PC, Chan AW, Li MK, Chan HY, et al. Disease progression of non-alcoholic fatty liver disease: A prospective study with paired liver biopsies at 3 years. Gut. 2010;**59**(7):969-974

[3] McPherson S, Hardy T, Henderson E, Burt AD, Day CP, Anstee QM. Evidence of NAFLD progression from steatosis to fibrosing-steatohepatitis using paired biopsies: Implications for prognosis and clinical management. Journal of Hepatology. 2015;**62**(5):1148-1155

[4] Ekstedt M, Franzen LE, Mathiesen UL, Thorelius L, Holmqvist M, Bodemar G, et al. Long-term follow-up of patients with NAFLD and elevated liver enzymes. Hepatology. 2006;**44**(4):865-873

[5] Calzadilla Bertot L, Adams LA. The natural course of non-alcoholic fatty liver disease. International Journal of Molecular Science. 2016;**17**:5

[6] Singh S, Allen AM, Wang Z, Prokop LJ, Murad MH, Loomba R. Fibrosis progression in nonalcoholic fatty liver vs nonalcoholic steatohepatitis: A systematic review and meta-analysis of paired-biopsy studies. Clinical Gastroenterology and Hepatology. 2015;**13**:643

[7] Pais R, Charlotte F, Fedchuk L, Bedossa P, Lebray P, Poynard T, et al. A systematic review of follow-up biopsies reveals disease progression in patients with non-alcoholic fatty liver. Journal of Hepatology. 2013;**59**(3):550-556

[8] Ward ZJ, Bleich SN, Cradock AL, Barrett JL, Giles CM, Flax C, et al. Projected U.S. State-level prevalence of adult obesity and severe obesity. The New England Journal of Medicine. 2019;**381**(25):2440-2450

[9] Estes C, Razavi H, Loomba R, Younossi Z, Sanyal AJ. Modeling the epidemic of nonalcoholic fatty liver disease demonstrates an exponential increase in burden of disease. Hepatology. 2018;**67**(1):123-133

[10] Lee SS, Park SH, Kim HJ, Kim SY, Kim M-Y, Kim DY, et al. Non-invasive assessment of hepatic steatosis: Prospective comparison of the accuracy of imaging examinations. Journal of Hepatology. 2010;**52**(4):579-585

[11] Hernaez R, Lazo M, Bonekamp S, Kamel I, Brancati FL, Guallar E, et al. Diagnostic accuracy and reliability of ultrasonography for the detection of fatty liver: A meta-analysis. Hepatology. 2011;**54**(3):1082-1090

[12] Ballestri S, Nascimbeni F, Baldelli E, Marrazzo A, Romagnoli D, Targher G, et al. Ultrasonographic fatty liver indicator detects mild steatosis and correlates with metabolic/histological parameters in various liver diseases. Metabolism. 2017;**72**:57-65

[13] Saadeh S, Younossi ZM, Remer EM, Gramlich T, Ong JP, Hurley M, et al. The utility of radiological imaging in nonalcoholic fatty liver disease. Gastroenterology. 2002;**123**(3):745-750

[14] Talwalkar JA, Kurtz DM, Schoenleber SJ, West CP, Montori VM. Ultrasound-based transient elastography for the detection of hepatic fibrosis: Systematic review and meta-analysis.

Clinical Gastroenterology and Hepatology. 2007;**5**(10):1214-1220

[15] Noureddin M, Lam J, Peterson MR, Middleton M, Hamilton G, Le T-A, et al. Utility of magnetic resonance imaging versus histology for quantifying changes in liver fat in nonalcoholic fatty liver disease trials. Hepatology. 2013;**58**(6):1930-1940

[16] Zhang B, Ding F, Chen T, Xia L-H, Qian J, Lv G-Y. Ultrasound hepatic/renal ratio and hepatic attenuation rate for quantifying liver fat content. World Journal of Gastroenterology. 2014;**20**(47):17985-17992

[17] Loomba R, Wolfson T, Ang B, Hooker J, Behling C, Peterson M, et al. Magnetic resonance elastography predicts advanced fibrosis in patients with nonalcoholic fatty liver disease: A prospective study. Hepatology. 2014;**60**(6):1920-1928

[18] Ioannou GN. Epidemiology and risk-stratification of NAFLD-associated HCC. Journal of Hepatology. 2021;**75**(6):1476-1484

[19] Kawamura Y, Arase Y, Ikeda K, Seko Y, Imai N, Hosaka T, et al. Large-Scale Long-Term Follow-Up Study of Japanese patients with non-alcoholic fatty liver disease for the onset of hepatocellular carcinoma. The American Journal of Gastroenterology. 2012;**107**(2):253-261

[20] Kanwal F, Kramer JR, Mapakshi S, Natarajan Y, Chayanupatkul M, Richardson PA, et al. Risk of hepatocellular cancer in patients with non-alcoholic fatty liver disease. Gastroenterology. 2018;**155**(6):1828

[21] Sørensen HT, Mellemkjaer L, Jepsen P, Thulstrup AM, Baron J, Olsen JH, et al. Risk of cancer in patients hospitalized with fatty liver: A Danish cohort study. Journal of Clinical Gastroenterology. 2003;**36**(4):356-359

[22] White DL, Kanwal F. Association between nonalcoholic fatty liver disease and risk for hepatocellular cancer, based on systematic review. Clinical Gastroenterology and Hepatology. 2012;**10**(12):1342

[23] Younossi Z, Stepanova M, Ong JP, Jacobson IM, Bugianesi E, Duseja A, et al. Nonalcoholic steatohepatitis is the fastest growing cause of hepatocellular carcinoma in liver transplant candidates. Clinical Gastroenterology and Hepatology. 2019;**17**(4):748

[24] Younossi ZM, Koenig AB, Abdelatif D, Fazel Y, Henry L, Wymer M. Global epidemiology of nonalcoholic fatty liver disease-Meta-analytic assessment of prevalence, incidence, and outcomes. Hepatology. 2016;**64**(1):73-84

[25] Bhaskaran K, Dos-Santos-Silva I, Leon DA, Douglas IJ, Smeeth L. Association of BMI with overall and cause-specific mortality: A population-based cohort study of 3·6 million adults in the UK. The Lancet Diabetes and Endocrinology. 2018;**6**(12):944-953

[26] Yang JD, Ahmed F, Mara KC, Addissie BD, Allen AM, Gores GJ, et al. Diabetes is associated with increased risk of hepatocellular carcinoma in patients with cirrhosis from nonalcoholic fatty liver disease. Hepatology. 2020;**71**(3):907-916

[27] Welzel TM, Graubard BI, Zeuzem S, El-Serag HB, Davila JA, McGlynn KA. Metabolic syndrome increases the risk of primary liver cancer in the United States: A study in the SEER-Medicare database. Hepatology. 2011;**54**(2):463-471

[28] Williams CD, Stengel J, Asike MI, Torres DM, Shaw J, Contreras M, et al. Prevalence of nonalcoholic fatty liver disease and nonalcoholic steatohepatitis among a largely middle-aged population utilizing ultrasound and liver biopsy: A prospective study. Gastroenterology. 2011;**140**(1):124-131

[29] Rich NE, Hester C, Odewole M, Murphy CC, Parikh ND, Marrero JA, et al. Racial and ethnic differences in presentation and outcomes of hepatocellular carcinoma. Clinical Gastroenterology and Hepatology. 2019;**17**(3):551

[30] Liu YL, Patman GL, Leathart JB, Piguet AC, Burt AD, Dufour JF, et al. Carriage of the PNPLA3 rs738409 C >G polymorphism confers an increased risk of non-alcoholic fatty liver disease associated hepatocellular carcinoma. Journal of Hepatology. 2014;**61**(1):75-81

[31] Anstee QM, Reeves HL, Kotsiliti E, Govaere O, Heikenwalder M. From NASH to HCC: Current concepts and future challenges. Nature Reviews. Gastroenterology & Hepatology. 2019;**16**(7):411-428

[32] Marra F, Svegliati-Baroni G. Lipotoxicity and the gut-liver axis in NASH pathogenesis. Journal of Hepatology. 2018;**68**(2):280-295

[33] Hatting M, Tacke F. From NAFLD to HCC: Is IL-17 the crucial link? Hepatology. 2017;**65**(2):739-741

[34] Huang DQ, El-Serag HB, Loomba R. Global epidemiology of NAFLD-related HCC: Trends, predictions, risk factors and prevention. Nature Reviews. Gastroenterology & Hepatology. 2021;**18**(4):223-238

[35] Pinyol R, Torrecilla S, Wang H, Montironi C, Pique-Gili M, Torres-Martin M, et al. Molecular characterisation of hepatocellular carcinoma in patients with non-alcoholic steatohepatitis. Journal of Hepatology. 2021;**75**(4):865-878

[36] Day CP, James OF. Steatohepatitis: A tale of two "hits"? Gastroenterology. 1998;**114**(4):842-845

[37] Lambert JE, Ramos-Roman MA, Browning JD, Parks EJ. Increased de novo lipogenesis is a distinct characteristic of individuals with nonalcoholic fatty liver disease. Gastroenterology. 2014;**146**(3):726-735

[38] Sunny NE, Bril F, Cusi K. Mitochondrial adaptation in nonalcoholic fatty liver disease: Novel mechanisms and treatment strategies. Trends in Endocrinology and Metabolism. 2017;**28**(4):250-260

[39] Sydor S, Best J, Messerschmidt I, Manka P, Vilchez-Vargas R, Brodesser S, et al. Altered microbiota diversity and bile acid signaling in cirrhotic and noncirrhotic NASH-HCC. Clinical and Translational Gastroenterology. 2020;**11**(3):e00131

[40] Yu YC, Luu HN, Wang R, Thomas CE, Glynn NW, Youk AO, et al. Serum biomarkers of iron status and risk of hepatocellular carcinoma development in patients with nonalcoholic fatty liver disease. Cancer Epidemiology, Biomarkers & Prevention. 2022;**31**(1):230-235

[41] Ringelhan M, Pfister D, O'Connor T, Pikarsky E, Heikenwalder M. The immunology of hepatocellular carcinoma. Nature Immunology. 2018;**19**(3):222-232

[42] Luther J, Garber JJ, Khalili H, Dave M, Bale SS, Jindal R, et al. Hepatic injury in nonalcoholic steatohepatitis contributes to altered intestinal

permeability. Cellular and Molecular Gastroenterology and Hepatology. 2015;**1**(2):222-232

[43] Ehling J, Bartneck M, Wei X, Gremse F, Fech V, Mockel D, et al. CCL2-dependent infiltrating macrophages promote angiogenesis in progressive liver fibrosis. Gut. 2014;**63**(12):1960-1971

[44] Lei L, Ei Mourabit H, Housset C, Cadoret A, Lemoinne S. Role of angiogenesis in the pathogenesis of NAFLD. Journal of Clinical Medicine. 2021;**10**(7):1960-1971

[45] Cabia B, Andrade S, Carreira MC, Casanueva FF, Crujeiras AB. A role for novel adipose tissue-secreted factors in obesity-related carcinogenesis. Obesity Reviews. 2016;**17**(4):361-376

[46] Carlessi R, Kohn-Gaone J, Olynyk JK, Tirnitz-Parker JEE. Mouse models of hepatocellular carcinoma. In: Tirnitz-Parker JEE, editor. Hepatocellular Carcinoma. Brisbane (AU): Codon Publications; 2019

[47] Tanaka S, Miyanishi K, Kobune M, Kawano Y, Hoki T, Kubo T, et al. Increased hepatic oxidative DNA damage in patients with nonalcoholic steatohepatitis who develop hepatocellular carcinoma. Journal of Gastroenterology. 2013;**48**(11):1249-1258

[48] Nishida N, Yada N, Hagiwara S, Sakurai T, Kitano M, Kudo M. Unique features associated with hepatic oxidative DNA damage and DNA methylation in non-alcoholic fatty liver disease. Journal of Gastroenterology and Hepatology. 2016;**31**(9):1646-1653

[49] Cornell L, Munck JM, Alsinet C, Villanueva A, Ogle L, Willoughby CE, et al. DNA-PK-A candidate driver of hepatocarcinogenesis and tissue biomarker that predicts response to treatment and survival. Clinical Cancer Research. 2015;**21**(4):925-933

[50] Zucman-Rossi J, Villanueva A, Nault JC, Llovet JM. Genetic landscape and biomarkers of hepatocellular carcinoma. Gastroenterology. 2015;**149**(5):1226

[51] European Association for the Study of the Liver. Electronic address eee, European Association for the Study of the L. EASL Clinical Practice Guidelines: Management of hepatocellular carcinoma. Journal of Hepatology. 2018;**69**(1):182-236

[52] Foerster F, Gairing SJ, Müller L, Galle PR. NAFLD-driven HCC: Safety and efficacy of current and emerging treatment options. Journal of Hepatology. 2022;**76**(2):446-457

[53] Llovet JM, Ricci S, Mazzaferro V, Hilgard P, Gane E, Blanc J-F, et al. Sorafenib in advanced hepatocellular carcinoma. The New England Journal of Medicine. 2008;**359**(4):378-390

[54] Cheng A-L, Kang Y-K, Chen Z, Tsao C-J, Qin S, Kim JS, et al. Efficacy and safety of sorafenib in patients in the Asia-Pacific region with advanced hepatocellular carcinoma: A phase III randomised, double-blind, placebo-controlled trial. The Lancet Oncology. 2009;**10**(1):25-34

[55] Bruix J, Raoul J-L, Sherman M, Mazzaferro V, Bolondi L, Craxi A, et al. Efficacy and safety of sorafenib in patients with advanced hepatocellular carcinoma: Subanalyses of a phase III trial. Journal of Hepatology. 2012;**57**(4):821-829

[56] Bruix J, Cheng A-L, Meinhardt G, Nakajima K, De Sanctis Y, Llovet J. Prognostic factors and predictors of

sorafenib benefit in patients with hepatocellular carcinoma: Analysis of two phase III studies. Journal of Hepatology. 2017;**67**(5):999-1008

[57] Howell J, Samani A, Mannan B, Hajiev S, Aval LM, Abdelmalak R, et al. Impact of NAFLD on clinical outcomes in hepatocellular carcinoma treated with sorafenib: An international cohort study. JCO. 2021;**39**(3):289

[58] Kudo M, Finn RS, Qin S, Han K-H, Ikeda K, Piscaglia F, et al. Lenvatinib versus sorafenib in first-line treatment of patients with unresectable hepatocellular carcinoma: A randomised phase 3 non-inferiority trial. The Lancet. 2018;**391**(10126):1163-1173

[59] Hiraoka A, Kumada T, Tada T, Tani J, Kariyama K, Fukunishi S, et al. Efficacy of lenvatinib for unresectable hepatocellular carcinoma based on background liver disease etiology: Multi-center retrospective study. Scientific Reports. 2021;**11**(1):16663

[60] Bruix J, Qin S, Merle P, Granito A, Huang Y-H, Bodoky G, et al. Regorafenib for patients with hepatocellular carcinoma who progressed on sorafenib treatment (RESORCE): A randomised, double-blind, placebo-controlled, phase 3 trial. The Lancet. 2017;**389**(10064):56-66

[61] Zhu AX, Park JO, Ryoo B-Y, Yen C-J, Poon R, Pastorelli D, et al. Ramucirumab versus placebo as second-line treatment in patients with advanced hepatocellular carcinoma following first-line therapy with sorafenib (REACH): A randomised, double-blind, multicentre, phase 3 trial. The Lancet Oncology. 2015;**16**(7):859-870

[62] Abou-Alfa GK, Meyer T, Cheng A-L, El-Khoueiry AB, Rimassa L, Ryoo B-Y, et al. Cabozantinib in patients with advanced and progressing hepatocellular carcinoma. The New England Journal of Medicine. 2018;**379**(1):54-63

[63] El-Khoueiry AB, Sangro B, Yau T, Crocenzi TS, Kudo M, Hsu C, et al. Nivolumab in patients with advanced hepatocellular carcinoma (CheckMate 040): An open-label, non-comparative, phase 1/2 dose escalation and expansion trial. Lancet. 2017;**389**(10088):2492-2502

[64] Zhu AX, Finn RS, Edeline J, Cattan S, Ogasawara S, Palmer D, et al. Pembrolizumab in patients with advanced hepatocellular carcinoma previously treated with sorafenib (KEYNOTE-224): A non-randomised, open-label phase 2 trial. The Lancet Oncology. 2018;**19**(7):940-952

[65] Finn RS, Ryoo B-Y, Merle P, Kudo M, Bouattour M, Lim HY, et al. Pembrolizumab as second-line therapy in patients with advanced hepatocellular carcinoma in KEYNOTE-240: A Randomized, Double-Blind, Phase III Trial. Journal of Clinical Oncology. 2020;**38**(3):193-202

[66] Yau T, Park J-W, Finn RS, Cheng A-L, Mathurin P, Edeline J, et al. Nivolumab versus sorafenib in advanced hepatocellular carcinoma (CheckMate 459): A randomised, multicentre, open-label, phase 3 trial. The Lancet Oncology. 2022;**23**(1):77-90

[67] Yau T, Kang Y-K, Kim T-Y, El-Khoueiry AB, Santoro A, Sangro B, et al. Efficacy and safety of nivolumab plus ipilimumab in patients with advanced hepatocellular carcinoma previously treated with sorafenib: The CheckMate 040 Randomized Clinical Trial. JAMA Oncology. 2020;**6**(11):e204564

[68] Dual Immunotherapy Makes Strides against HCC. Cancer Discovery. 2022;**12**(4). Available from:

https://aacrjournals.org/cancerdiscovery/article/12/4/OF1/689618/Dual-Immunotherapy-Makes-Strides-against-HCCDual

[69] Finn RS, Qin S, Ikeda M, Galle PR, Ducreux M, Kim T-Y, et al. Atezolizumab plus Bevacizumab in Unresectable Hepatocellular Carcinoma. The New England Journal of Medicine. 2020;**382**(20):1894-1905

[70] Pfister D, Nunez NG, Pinyol R, Govaere O, Pinter M, Szydlowska M, et al. NASH limits anti-tumour surveillance in immunotherapy-treated HCC. Nature. 2021;**592**(7854):450-456

Chapter 3

Hepatic Progression of Hepatocellular Carcinoma

Anna Rossetto, Alessandro Rosignoli, Brunilda Tatani, Valli De Re and Alessandro Uzzau

Abstract

Hepatocellular carcinoma constitutes an ongoing challenge due to its incidence and the high mortality related to it. Metastases and relapses even after treatment with curative intent are frequent. The liver is a common site for metastasis because of anatomical and physiological reasons; its position, the particular cytoarchitecture and cell populations, and its peculiar immunologic properties make it a favorable and tolerogenic environment; the inflammatory state with the alteration of the cytoarchitecture and of the microcirculation associated, and gut permeability and metabolic diseases cause the development of a liable site to progression of hepatocellular carcinoma. The difficulty of always having an early diagnosis and the lack of therapeutic flow charts including the biological behavior of the disease have always posed great difficulties in dealing with it. In the last few years, mechanisms involved in the onset and in the progression of hepatocellular carcinoma are a source of great interest; the discovery of pro-neoplastic and pro-metastatic conditions, of the cross talk between organs and cells, of progression pathways, of mediators contributing to proliferation and metastasis and of modular check points, of miRNAs, all potential therapeutic targets, appear promising for transforming the approach to hepatocarcinoma, offering the possibility of earlier diagnosis, customizable treatments, and better outcome.

Keywords: hepatocellular carcinoma, liver metastasis, hepatic progression of hepatocellular carcinoma, immunotolerance, ischemia/riperfusion injury, miRNAs

1. Introduction

Hepatocellular carcinoma (HCC) is the third leading cause of cancer-related death. Locoregional treatment, surgical resection, and liver transplantation are main and most efficient treatments, but the risks of recurrence and metastasis are very high (70% after primary liver resection with curative intent) [1].

The risk of recurrence in HCC is high because of the biological and morphological nature of the liver.

Recurrent disease includes both intrahepatic metastasis, which usually form within the first 2 years of diagnosis, and de novo cancer that generally occurs later. The hepatic vascular anatomy and immunological characteristics create a pro-neoplastic niche for metastasis, while the continuing damage to the liver creates pro-neoplastic sites susceptible to secondary tumors. Liver metastasis represents a big challenge in the battle against cancer because they have a high mortality rate. Around 30–70% of patients die with liver metastasis, and metastasis is responsible for more than 90% cancer mortality [1].

The position of liver, near the gastrointestinal tract, only partially justifies the metastasis toward it. In fact, for other types of "distant" cancer, the liver is the first and sometimes even the only target of metastasis (e.g., uveal melanoma and triple-negative breast cancer). This consequently suggests that the criterion of proximity is only partially a predisposing factor but rather that there are specific tumor and extra tumor elements that predispose to metastasization to the liver. Another factor that has emerged in recent years is the exchange of information and the "preconditioning" of the liver that occurs before the actual establishment of metastatic colonies.

However, the development of knowledge on the local and systemic factors that promote the advance of the neoplastic disease and favor its metastasis has thus highlighted multiple and rich pathways that are fascinating from a speculative point of view but above all promising for the development of future preventive and therapeutic strategies.

2. Peculiar liver characteristics

The liver is the only organ with double arterial and venous vascularization. It constitutes the first filter for all effluent blood from the gastrointestinal district. The cytoarchitecture with the lobular arrangement, the portal spaces, and the intricate network of discontinuous capillaries (sinusoids) constitutes a unique feature. Multiple cell populations with their pathophysiological implications are responsible of a myriad of actions including favoring or not, the development of metastases.

The cellular structure of the liver is composed of 70% hepatocytes and 30% from non-parenchymal cells, which are crucial in the activation of many very characteristic liver phenomena.

2.1 Hepatic stellate cells

In a physiological condition, the stellate cells represent 1.5% of the entire hepatic parenchyma and 1/3 of the non-parenchymal cell compartment. They have multiple functions, from the ability to store lipids and vitamin A, to their involvement in the reparative phenomena of the hepatic parenchyma, fibrinogenesis, and the maintenance of homeostasis. They have intrahepatic and subendothelial cytoplasmic extensions through which they can establish connections with hepatocytes; are sensitive to the chemotactic stimulus and respond to alpha adrenergic activation. They are activated following the inflammatory stimulus, losing their lipid vacuoles, and developing microfilaments evolving into myofibroblasts. They play a key role in fetal hepatic development, become fundamental in the phenomena of hepatic regeneration of the adult liver and in the remodeling of the extracellular matrix through the secretion of angiogenetic factors, cytokines (IL-6, IL-10, TGF-β), adhesion molecules, connective tissue growth factor (CTGF), Endothelin-1, contributing to the activation of endothelial cells and facilitating the extravasation of neoplastic cells in the liver and supporting metastasizing [1].

They can undergo the mesenchymal-to-epithelial transition and thus become liver progenitor cells giving rise to hepatocytes. They also play an important action at the immunological level as they can act as antigen receptor cells (APCs), receive stimuli from leukocytes, support leukocyte recruitment and activation, modulate the intensity of the activation of the immune response. They are the main cell type involved in fibrogenesis in response to liver damage [2].

2.2 Kupffer cells (KCs)

They represent 20–30% of non-parenchymal cells. They are liver-derived macrophages that support both innate and adaptive immune responses to pathogens originating from the gastrointestinal tract through the effluent blood arriving via the portal vein. They are activated through two types of polarization, classical (M1), when stimulated by IFN, TNF, GM-CSF, or mycrobic stimuli or alternative (M2) when stimulated by IL-4, IL-13 and IL-33. They perform important functions in the mechanism of liver damage, in ischemic/reperfusion injury, in alcoholic liver disease, in nonalcoholic fatty liver disease, in immunotolerance phenomena after liver transplantation, and in endotoxin tolerance modulation. In response to the inflammatory stimulus, they are involved in the activation of HSCs, thus promoting fibrosis through the release of mediators (TGF-beta and platelet-derived growth factor).

Hepatic sinusoid stromal cells, hepatic sinusoidal endothelial cells, and stellate cells are the first liver cells to come into contact with systemic antigens and derived from the gastrointestinal tract [1, 3, 4].

2.3 Immunotolerance

Another fundamental aspect is its function as a tolerogenic immunosuppressive organ toward the molecules absorbed by the intestine and therefore, at the same time, the tumor cells and infectious agents. The liver contains numerous immune system cells, both adaptive and innate, specialized in the recognition and capture of infectious agents with the recruitment of inflammatory and leukocyte cells and the presentation of antigens to lymphocytes in the bloodstream. However, this mechanism must be finely controlled so that the immune response is not implemented toward non-pathogenic molecules such as those of the host or deriving from ingested food. It is this balance between activation of the immune response and its inhibition characterizes the liver as the main organ of the host's first immune barrier [5–7].

The idea that the immune system plays an important role in the development of neoplastic pathology is dated and has been controversial for years; however, several studies on transplants have expanded knowledge about tolerance since the ability to induce tolerance toward the transplanted organ is essential for the survival of the graft.

While it is clear that through the oral route and the gastrointestinal system tolerance can be induced through the local activation of the gastrointestinal immune system, it is, however, shown that much of the induction of the tolerance process takes place in the liver. In particular, survival of the graft in liver transplantation has been demonstrated in subjects without kinship ties of some animal species without immunosuppression and still in some cases in which the expression of a tolerant phenotype allowed the suspension of immunosuppressive therapy [8, 9].

The hepatic parenchyma therefore has very important immunological functions and the peculiar ability to induce tolerance: the activation of the liver immune system, consisting of macrophages, dendritic cells, natural killer, and T lymphocytes, produces immunological mediators (in particular IL 10, TGF beta, and others), which, on the one hand, induce localized immunological suppression aimed at minimizing liver damage, on the other create a tolerant environment for the colonization of metastatic clones. Both sinusoidal endothelial cells and stellate cells activated by TGF-beta and PDGF are strongly involved in the maintenance of local and systemic tolerance phenomena. In addition, the same T lymphocytes made tolerant are then able to return to the primary tumor and suppress the local defense systems [6–12].

The involvement of the immune response and immunocompetence in the development of neoplastic diseases has been, and still is, a subject of debate, because many of the tumor antigens are self-antigens for which the immunological response is weaker and more difficult to measure. However, it is well known that individuals with a decline in immune defenses related to old age, or undergoing immunosuppressive therapies, or suffering from immune system disorders such as chronic infections or autoimmune diseases have an increased risk for the development of metaplasia; even the most common and recognized risk factors for cancers such as smoking, alcohol abuse, advanced age, and poor nutritional status are associated with more or less pronounced alterations of the immune system and risk of metastasis [13].

2.4 Cancer-derived microvescicles

Cancer-derived microvesicles have recently been identified as responsible for very important roles at the level of the tumor microenvironment, contributing through their load to the development of metastases and to the selection of organotropism. The microvesicles produced by the tumor cells are released into the circulation before the cancer cells reach metastatic sites.

The information transmitted by them is able to initiate a congenial soil phenomenon (as claimed in Paget's theory) starting processes of angiogenesis, cancer-associated fibroblasts (CAFs) formation, endothelial cell migration.

The signal mediated by microvesicles allows an exchange of intracellular information with the possibility of modulating the migratory and metastatic behavior of more quiescent cells but also of inducing drug resistance. They are also able to reduce the immune response by increasing the development of immunosuppressive cell populations (PD-1 positive nonclassical monocyte) reprogram the cellular metabolism of neoplastic cells, which is a fundamental step in the extravasation and dissemination of tumor cells.

In the studies of the last few years, it appears increasingly evident that the target organs for the development of metastases undergo phenomena that define their receptivity and mediated by the primary tumor well before the development of metastases.

At the hepatic level, the extracellular vesicles produced by the neoplastic cells first interface with the Kupffer cells. The information deriving from the EVs affects the hepatic stromal cells with the consequent activation of hepatocyte growth factor, which favors the development of fertile soil for the development of metastases [14–17].

3. Metastasis mechanisms, seed and soil theory

The establishment of metastatic colonies requires a complex network of interactions with the microenvironment consisting of extracellular matrix, stromal and inflammatory cells, vessels.

The first and well-known theory on the mechanisms of development of metastases dates back more than a century with the beautiful metaphor of Paget in his concept of seed and soil theory. In a study resulting from the metastatic spread of breast cancer, he compared the tumor to a plant that spreads its seeds everywhere; however, the seeds can germinate and grow only where they find the suitable soil.

Subsequently, other scholars have tried to explain the phenomenon by attributing its origin mainly to anatomical and hemodynamic factors (p.e. J.Edwing). With current knowledge, this provides only a small piece of the complex phenomenon of metastatic advancement and organotropism. We know that there are specific factors of the tumor but also systemic and specific factors of the target organs that determine the evolution of the neoplastic disease. The study of these phenomena is extremely current and promising since metastatic cancer continues to support a very large percentage of deaths and therefore remains an open challenge of fundamental importance [18]. Local phenomena, systemic phenomena, and specific target organ phenomena that are responsible for the advancement and spread of the disease have been identified. Starting from the local phenomena that are characteristic of the neoplastic and peri-neoplastic tissue (but in reality also involved at the level of distant organs site of metastases), we consider the metabolic alterations and the consequent reduction of pH. In fact, it is now a historical acquisition, the condition for which neoplastic cells use a huge amount of glucose to maintain their proliferation generating a large amount of lactic acid as a waste product. This in turn leads to a decrease in pH in the extracellular space with the onset of a condition of acidosis in the tumor microenvironment. This is known as the Warburg effect.

If acidosis by itself favors processes such as metastasis, angiogenesis, and immunosuppression, and given the coexistence of areas with different tumor metabolism (areas closer to the vessels, more oxygenated and farther, more hypoxic), the high concentration of lactates allows phenomena of metabolic adaptation such as "metabolic symbiosis" and "reverse Warburg effect," improving the survival of the neoplastic cells [19].

The local immunological response (cancer immunoediting) plays another fundamental function in allowing neoplastic progression to metastatic disease and is also closely linked to local metabolic and hypoxic phenomena. This concept has appeared of great interest in recent years in view of the therapeutic repercussions that are due to immunotherapy introduction.

This phenomenon is summarized in three steps: the elimination (the first step) of the neoplastic cells by the immune system, the balance (the second step), that is, the moment in which the two systems (neoplasm and organism) are apparently balanced, and finally, the tumor escape when a situation is established in which the immunological response is overcome [20]. Some chemokines, produced in response to inflammatory stimuli of the peritumoral zone, attract leukocytes (polymorphonuclear neutrophils) to the sites of inflammation and play an important role in the homing and proliferation of cancer cells, representing an important component of the phenomenon of escape from the unfavorable environment of primitive cancer cells. However, the classic concept of peri-neoplastic inflammatory tissue with pro-tumoral activities has undergone conceptual evolutions with the definition of an immunological threshold beyond which the normally tumorigenic phenomenon becomes rather beneficial by developing the idea of an intensification of the local inflammatory stimulus can be exploited in therapeutic terms [10–12, 21].

4. Liver diseases and hepatocellular carcinoma progression

The process of metastasis is a complex phenomenon that occurs through multiple steps, from intravasation after the escape from the primary tumor, to the overcoming of the systems of recognition and cellular destruction, to the invasion and survival in the blood stream. Cells that manage to overcome these steps have developed a high capacity for metastasis through accumulation of genetic and epigenetic alterations including microRNA (miRNA) expression changes.

In HCC, venous metastases develop through dissemination by portal and through the formation of neoplastic thrombi by neoplastic cells that have acquired the molecular changes that allow them to survive and invade the venous stream [22].

Hypoxia is common to many tumors. In HCC, hypoxia is present and responsible of progression and metastatization.

Liver cirrhosis and the rapid growth of the neoplastic nodule determine a reduction in blood flow with the consequent establishment of a hypoxic state. Both liver cirrhosis and tumor size (>8 cm) are independent risk factors for development of portal vein tumor thrombi. PVTT is present in 20–70% of HCC and correlates with poor prognosis.

Under hypoxia conditions, the expression of 14-3-3ζ is increased, which induced hypoxia-induced factor-1α (HIF-1α) expression by stabilizing HIF-1α protein. This resulted in an enhanced EMT response of HCC cells, promoting the formation of PVTT and HCC metastasis.

Both HIF-1α levels and PVTT formation in HCC are strongly correlated with 14-3-3ζ expression [23].

During the metastasis process, the biological characteristics of the target organs are decisive. Generally, the target organs, already in the initial state of the disease, even before the onset of metastases, have already been affected by factors deriving from the primary tumor. Furthermore, the metastatic microenvironment does not depend only on the anatomy and biology of the target organ but also on the pathophysiological phenomena altered by the products of neoplastic cells or by preexisting conditions. Numerous studies have evaluated the implications of a preexisting liver disease or chronic inflammatory condition on the evolution of the development of metastases with sometimes conflicting results [24–28]. The coexistence of a preexisting inflammatory activation, the presence of a subversion of the parenchymal structure, an alteration of the extracellular matrix, the activation of stellate and Kupffer cells, and the condition of oxidative stress that is created are phenomena that are recognized responsible in the promotion of metastasis [1, 29–32].

Given its double vascularization with a much higher venous supply, it is mainly a hypoxic microenvironment [33].

If on the one hand, the frequent metastasis to the liver depends on its peculiar characteristics of the microcirculation and sinusoidal permeability and on the physiologically immunotolerant environment that distinguishes it, on the other hand, the neoplastic cells to constitute metastatic colonies enter into "metabolic" competition with normal liver cells precisely because of the hypoxic environment and learn to "mimic" the metabolic behavior of normal liver cells.

Recent studies have demonstrated the ability of an epigenetic remodeling, which, through enhancers or super enhancers, can modify the specific transcription program of circulating tumor cells (specific to the tumor type) by making them acquire a liver-specific transcription program [34].

The molecular mechanisms that metastatic cells have acquired to obviate the metabolic problems deriving from the hypoxic environment, that is, different according to the tumor type, have also been described.

The activation of intrahepatic cells can modify the metabolic behavior of metastatic cells. In particular, stellate cells, normally quiescent, when activated in a context that from poorly inflammatory becomes inflammatory can affect their metabolic state, proliferation ability, and stem cell characteristics.

Also ketone bodies metabolism, enterohepatic circulation of bile acid, and ammonia metabolism may change the metabolic behavior of cancer cells, since neoplastic cells are also able to use waste products that hepatocytes cannot use, to generate energy, thanks to their marked ability to adapt, confirming how their metabolism is anything but a static phenomenon. These alternative pathways are therefore also able to determine activation of quiescientious cells [35].

However, it is essential to consider the complexity, bidirectionality, and specificity of this whole cascade of events. In fact, the systemic repercussions, which occur from the beginning of the onset of neoplastic pathology, presuppose a two-way communication between neoplasm and host with the establishment of both protumor and antitumor pathways; moreover they are patient-specific, dependent on the specific patient's background and on the coexistence of different pathophysiological conditions including comorbidities and ongoing therapy; similarly the metastatic potential of circulating cancer cells is extremely heterogeneous from patient to patient.

4.1 Ischemia/reperfusion injury, gut-liver axis, and angiogenesis

Ischemia/reperfusion damage (IRI) is a well-known para-physiological phenomenon that follows hepatic surgical resection and transplantation procedures. It's is commonly interpreted as a state of sterile inflammation. After ischemic state is established, the liver tissue initiates a cascade of events leading to hepatocellular injury, alteration of liver function, and worsened oncological outcomes in the presence of cancer [36].

After a time of iatrogenic ischemia induced by clamping the portal peduncle to limit blood losses or necessary for the packaging of vascular anastomoses, the restoration of perfusion causes a cascade of inflammatory and repair phenomena.

If during the ischemia phase, the cells are subjected to hypoxic stress with a decrease in pH, ATP depletion, accumulation of intracellular Ca, and activation of various forms of cellular death, then with the reperfusion phase there is the formation of reactive oxygen species (ROS), activation of the immunological response, release of chemokines and inflammatory cytokines, of cell damage mediating molecules (DAMPs), and activation of hepatic cellular subpopulations.

In this circumstance, through the phenomenon of immune escape and neo-angiogenesis promoted by the cascade of events resulting from IRI, the risk of recurrence and disease progression makes its way.

At the same time, the portal clamping causes a venous congestion of the gastrointestinal tract with hypoperfusion and subsequent establishment of mucosal damage that determines an alteration of permeability with subsequent bacterial translocation. Ischemia/reperfusion damage and increased intestinal permeability are related to a risk of recurrence both after transplantation and after liver resection due to the onset of exacerbated inflammation.

Therefore, the modulation of the inflammatory response and the modulation of the gut-liver axis prove to be key points on which to act to reduce the oncological risk.

Steatotic livers are more sensitive to damage from ischemia/reperfusion due to alterations in the microcirculation caused by the accumulation of lipids with a consequent decrease in the sinusoidal space and because of a lower amount of stored energy and a greater sensitivity of the cell membrane to lipid peroxidation caused by ischemia/reperfusion. The same applies to aged livers: are much more sensitive to ischemia/reperfusion damage [37].

Recently it has been observed that small for size syndrome is also involved as a negative prognostic factor after liver surgery in terms of risk of recurrence for HCC. It constitutes a postsurgical complication with hepatic insufficiency and due to its analogy with the damage induced by the phenomenon of ischemia/reperfusion, it also causes mechanical damage in the acute phase, in fact, highlighting a correspondence between parenchymal liver damage and the possibility of implantation of circulating neoplastic cells.

Moreover, it has been seen that these acute-phase phenomena not only favor the implantation of neoplastic cells for factors related to the other microcirculation and the inflammatory cascade but also are able to modify the behavior of neoplastic cells favoring their aggressiveness by directly activating cell migration and invasion pathways [37].

Promising strategies to reduce this risk are normothermic or hypothermic oxygenated perfusions aimed at reducing oxidative stress especially when the graft is suboptimal and is therefore even more sensitive to the cascade of inflammatory phenomena triggered by IRI.

Changes in iatrogenically induced ischemia during hepatic resection have also been explored in order to reduce intraoperative bleeding such as selective portal clamping, maintaining arterial flow, and remote ischemic preconditioning. These strategies appear to reduce ischemia/reperfusion damage resulting in a positive effect in terms of the risk of HCC recurrence [38].

4.2 Renin-angiotensin system

The renin-angiotensin system seems to be involved in multiple aspects of the evolution of HCC and in the development of metastases. Overexpressions of components of this axis in hepatocarcinoma have been highlighted. In addition, its components are able to promote cell proliferation, angiogenesis, extracellular matrix formation, and fibrosis progression; they can interact with the m-TOR pathway and inhibit apoptosis.

They promote fibrosis: some components of the renin-angiotensin axis are able to modulate liver fibrosis through the activation of HSCs and the deposition of extracellular matrix; treatment with Losartan as a pharmacological agent active on angiotensin II receptors is able to reduce liver fibrosis.

They stimulate neo-angiogenesis by modulation of growth factors such as VEGF and TGF-beta, promoting epithelium-mesenchymal transition, inducing the formation of reactive oxygen species (classical pathway) or through the activation of non-classical TGF-beta/MAPK pathway involvement of apoptotic, metabolic, and cell proliferation phenomena [39].

The mechanisms involved are:

- Activation of AT1R promoting cell proliferation, inflammation, angiogenesis, and extracellular matrix formation while Mas receptor (MasR), other component of RAS, has a protective role since it inhibits the effects of AT1R.

- Phosphoinositide 3-kinase (PI3K)/AKT/mammalian target of rapamycin (mTOR) pathway promotes HCC cell proliferation and inhibits apoptosis, and the RAS system reduces the survival rate of HCC patients by mediating PI3K/AKT/mTOR pathway.

- Ang II induces vascular endothelial growth factor (VEGF) and transforming growth factor-β (TGF-β) to promote angiogenesis and aggravate liver fibrosis, respectively.

4.3 Insulin resistance and diabetes type 2

Insulin resistance and diabetes type 2 are involved in the onset and progression of hepatocellular carcinoma.

In chronic liver disease generally underlying the onset of HCC, there are conditions of insulin resistance and type 2 diabetes linked to obesity and dyslipidemia but also diabetes of hepatic origin caused by HCV, alcohol intake, structural alterations, reduction in liver mass with consequent reduction of insulin clearance by Kupffer cells and endothelial cells or by constitution of collateral circles following portal hypertension with the establishment of shunts and therefore bypassing the hepatic extraction.

All these conditions lead to increased blood insulin levels. An excess of insulin in blood dictated by resistance to it determines secretion at the hepatic level of insulin-like growth factor (known to stimulate cellular proliferation and also inhibit apoptosis within the liver) [40].

A situation of insulin resistance is established following hyperinsulinemia due to the consequent downregulation of IRs, i.e., reduced receptor affinity, reduced availability at target, and a reduced efficacy, due to increase in glucagon, growth hormone, IGF, free fatty acids, and cytokines [41, 42].

Diabetes mellitus (DM) is identified as a negative prognostic indicator in hepatocellular carcinoma (HCC) since it has been shown to be associated with significantly higher incidence of histological macrovascular invasion and a higher rate of distant metastatic disease [43].

4.4 Cancer stem cells, down- or upregulated pathways, driving genes and epigenetic modifications

During the inflammatory and regenerative state that determines the development and progression of hepatocarcinoma, many events take place including the expansion of stem cells, the modification of the microenvironment as well as the multiple genetic and epigenetic changes that give the neoplastic cells the ability to survive and proliferate. Organogenesis and the development of a hepatic neoplasm are similar phenomena.

In both cases, cell proliferation, angiogenesis, and cross talk phenomena with the microenvironment occur.

Cancer stem cells are tumorigenic and metastatic and are markedly elevated in chronic liver diseases; hepatocytes, in these conditions have lost part of their proliferative capacity. This causes the expansion of stem cells (ductular reactions). The self-renewal, differentiation, proliferation, survival, angiogenesis, and migration of CSCs in several malignancies are promoted by the Notch signaling pathway.

To obtain tumor regression, eradication of cancer stem cells is considered sufficient. This has an important implication from the point of view of therapeutic application as the eradication of cancer stem cells could determine the regression of the neoplasm [44].

The acquisition of changes in the upregulation or downregulation of progression pathways (EGFR, Ras/Raf/Erk, PI3/Akt/mTOR, JAK, Shp2,..) is a phenomenon that allows the progression of the disease and that determines the development of resistance or poor efficacy of pharmacological therapies.

This suggests on the one hand the need to identify the type of HCC on the basis of the expression of these alterations as it results in a prognostic stratification based on the expected response to therapy, and on the other hand, it offers the possibility of studying personalized therapeutic combinations aimed at improving the outcome by acting on the molecular path that determines the response.

The introduction of therapies for advanced HCC not susceptible to surgical therapy (multikinase inhibitors) has made it possible to expand the therapeutic possibilities thanks to the discovery of new therapeutic targets but also has shown a great heterogenicity of response and high levels of resistances that require customization therapeutic strategies [45].

Tumorigenesis and tumor progression are promoted by genetic and epigenetic changes. This makes it possible to overcome immunological barriers, to survive changes in the environment, pH, and metabolism, to acquire the ability to metastasize and to acquire resistance to therapies.

Alterations that commonly occur in HCC have been highlighted:

- CTNNB1-related WNT-beta-catenin and most commonly present in HCV-related liver disease;

- VEGFA and IGF2, which promote neoplastic progression and angiogenesis.

- KRAS, quite infrequent in HCC but closely related to MKI resistance.

Each of these alterations constitutes a possible therapeutic window; the inhibition of Wnt/β-catenin pathway determines a reduction in the phenomenon of epithelial mesenchymal transition and increases radiosensitivity.

Several specific molecular targets for antiangiogenic agents are being explored; sorafenib, exerts antiangiogenic effects through VEGF receptor (VEGFR) and platelet-derived growth factor receptor (PDGFR) inhibition [46].

4.5 miRNA

MicroRNAs are small single-strand non-coding of about 22 nucleotides in length.

MicroRNAs binds to complementary sequences of target mRNA and performs the posttrascriptional regulatory activity; each miRNA can target hundreds of mRNA.

They are important regulatory molecules in gene expression processes. miRNAs are involved in physiological and pathological processes and play different roles in carcinogenesis processes, progression, invasion, metastatization, cell cycle, apoptosis, and drug resistance. Some miRNAs are involved in modulating epithelial-mesenchymal transition through downregulation of E-cadherin, enhancing HCC metastasis, and some are involved in PVTT formation determining high level of TGF beta and favoring immune escape.

They have a dual role: in HCC some miRNAs are overexpressed, others are downregulated, suggesting they can act as oncogenic factor or as tumor suppressor.

microRNAs also play pivotal roles in immune-modulation and antitumor immunity [47–50].

The cross talk between epigenetics and miRNA is important in the molecular pathogenesis of HCC: some studies demonstrate that epigenetic alteration can silence miRNAs with tumor suppressor activities.

Restoring the expression of tumor suppressor miRNA could be used for cancer treatment [51].

The molecular heterogeneity of HCC indeed still represents a critical factor; some microRNAs are associated with HCC or related to HCC subtypes, suggesting the potential role of microRNAs for HCC patient stratification terms of diagnosis and prognosis but also in the allocation of the best therapeutic plan with the potential for personalized adjuvant therapy; miRNAs are promising tools also as molecular biomarkers (both tissue and circulating) to predict mestastasis and postsurgical recurrence as well as therapeutic targets [52].

From the therapeutic point of view, the possibility to use miRNA looks very promising: there are studies on the silencing of "oncogenic" miRNAs through the endovenous administration of antagonists, on miRNA restoration, of those with onco-suppressive function, through administration by adeno-associated virus or non-viral miRNA delivery system [52].

5. Conclusions

The treatment of HCC poses a great challenge due to the high incidence, high mortality rate caused by relapses after treatment. For years many classifications have followed one another in order to try to standardize the treatment based on the stage of the disease to obtain the best possible benefit. However, an insufficient definition of the stratification caused by the heterogeneity of the biological behavior and also of the patient's response has always emerged. The absence of biomarkers indicative of the degree of aggression and the biological features has always placed a major limitation causing "blind spots" at the time of therapeutic choice.

Furthermore, due to the very nature of the disease and the general conditions of the patient, the diagnosis is often made late or the surgical possibilities are not feasible. The study and discovery of the steps of carcinogenesis and of the phenomena involved in the progression of the disease are of great interest and have provided fundamental elements for the treatment (with the introduction of new therapeutic substances starting from MK inhibitors to miRNA or immunoterapies).

Thanks to the discovery of pathways and checkpoints, essential steps for the rise and progression of HCC, many therapeutic strategies have been studied with the aim of blocking a certain "step" or even reprogramming the aggression and the ability to metastasize or to modulate the resistance/sensitivity to therapies. The introduction of biomarkers and diagnostic strategies such as liquid biopsy allows to carry out diagnostic studies in much earlier stages than in the past, overcoming problems of this disease in terms of seeding risk, inadequacy in describing phenomena of vascular invasion and biological aggression, or to dynamically monitor neoplastic progression.

The combination of these diagnostic tools and these therapeutic strategies seems extremely promising; they could substantially change the approach to HCC with early diagnosis and patient-tailored therapies.

Author details

Anna Rossetto[1*], Alessandro Rosignoli[2], Brunilda Tatani[2], Valli De Re[3] and Alessandro Uzzau[4]

1 General Surgery Unit, ASUFC, San Daniele del Friuli, Udine, Italy

2 Department General Surgery, Academical Hospital (ASUFC), Udine, Italy

3 Immunopatologia e Biomarcatori Oncologici/Bio-proteomics Facility, Centro di Riferimento Oncologico di Aviano (CRO), Italy

4 HPB Unit, Academical Hospital (ASUFC), Udine, Italy

*Address all correspondence to: anna.rossetto@asufc.sanita.fvg.it

References

[1] Rossetto A, De Re V, Steffan A, et al. Carcinogenesis and metastasis in liver: Cell physiological basis. Cancers (Basel). 2019;**11**:1731

[2] Sufleţel RT, Melincovici CS, Gheban BA, Toader Z, Mihu CM. Hepatic stellate cells—From past till present: Morphology, human markers, human cell lines, behavior in normal and liver pathology. Journal of Morphology and Embryology. 2020;**61**:615

[3] Li P, He K, Li J, Liu Z, Gong J. The role of Kupffer cells in hepatic diseases. Molecular Immunology. 2017;**85**:222-229

[4] Brenner C, Galluzzi L, Kepp O, Kroemer G. Decoding cell death signals in liver inflammation. Journal of Hepatology. 2013;**59**(3):583-594

[5] Vidal-Vanaclocha F. The liver prometastatic reaction of cancer patients: Implications for microenvironment-dependent colon cancer gene regulation. Cancer Microenvironment. 2011;**4**(2):163-180

[6] Nemeth E, Baird AW, O'Farrelly C. Microanatomy of the liver immune system. Seminars in Immunopathology. 2009;**31**(3):333-343

[7] Schildberg FA, Sharpe AH, Turley SJ. Hepatic immune regulation by stromal cells. Current Opinion in Immunology. 2015;**32**:1-6

[8] Starzl TE, Murase N, Abu-Elmagd K, Gray EA, Shapiro R, Eghtesad B, et al. Tolerogenic immunosuppression for organ transplantation. Lancet. 2003;**361**(9368):1502-1510

[9] Tiegs G, Lohse AW. Immune tolerance: What is unique about the liver. Journal of Autoimmunity. 2010;**34**(1):1-6

[10] Van den Eynden GG, Majeed AW, Illemann M, Vermeulen PB, Bird NC, Høyer-Hansen G, et al. The multifaceted role of the microenvironment in liver metastasis: Biology and clinical implications. Cancer Research. 2013;**73**(7):2031-2043

[11] Eveno C, Hainaud P, Rampanou A, Bonnin P, Bakhouche S, Dupuy E, et al. Proof of prometastatic niche induction by hepatic stellate cells. The Journal of Surgical Research. 2015;**194**(2):496-504

[12] Kang N, Gores GJ, Shah VH. Hepatic stellate cells: Partners in crime for liver metastases? Hepatology. 2011;**54**(2):707-713

[13] Jewell AP. Is the liver an important site for the development of immune tolerance to tumours? Medical Hypotheses. 2005;**64**(4):751-754

[14] Mo Z, Cheong JYA, Xiang L, Le MTN, Grimson A, Zhang DX. Extracellular vesicle-associated organotropic metastasis. Cell Proliferation. 2021;**54**(1):e12948

[15] Hoshino A, Costa-Silva B, Shen TL, Rodrigues G, Hashimoto A, Tesic Mark M, et al. Tumour exosome integrins determine organotropic metastasis. Nature. 2015;**527**(7578): 329-335

[16] Shao Y, Chen T, Zheng XI, et al. Colorectal cancer-derived small extracellular vesicles establish an inflammatory premetastatic niche in liver metastasis. Carcinogenesis. 2018;**39**(11):1368-1379

[17] Zhang H, Deng T, Liu R, et al. Exosome-delivered EGFR regulatesliver microenvironment to promote gastric

cancer liver metastasis. Nature Communications. 2017;**8**:15016

[18] Liu Q, Zhang H, Jiang X, et al. Factors involved in cancer metastasis: A better understanding to "seed and soil" hypothesis. Molecular Cancer. 2017;**16**:176

[19] de la Cruz-López KG et al. Lactate in the regulation of tumor microenvironment and therapeutic approaches. Frontiers in Oncology. 2019;**9**:1143

[20] Cruz-Bermúdez A, Laza-Briviesca R, Casarrubios M, Sierra-Rodero B, Provencio M. The role of metabolism in tumor immune evasion: Novel approaches to improve immunotherapy. Biomedicine. 2021;**9**(4):361

[21] Brú A, Gómez-Castro D, Vila L, Brú I, Souto JC. Study of tumor growth indicates the existence of an "immunological threshold" separating states of pro- and antitumoral peritumoral inflammation. PLoS One. 2018;**13**(11):e0202823. Published 2018 Nov 2. DOI: 10.1371/journal.pone.0202823

[22] Wong CM, Wong CC, Lee JM, Fan DN, Au SL, Ng IO. Sequential alterations of microRNA expression in hepatocellular carcinoma development and venous metastasis. Hepatology. 2012;**55**(5):1453-1461

[23] Tang Y, Liu S, Li N, Guo W, Shi J, Yu H, et al. 14-3-3ζ promotes hepatocellular carcinoma venous metastasis by modulating hypoxia-inducible factor-1α. Oncotarget. 2016;7(13):15854

[24] Augustin G, Bruketa T, Korolija D, Milosevic M. Lower incidence of hepatic metastases of colorectal cancer in patients with chronic liver diseases: Meta-analysis. Hepato-Gastroenterology. 2013;**60**(125):1164

[25] Wu W, Chen J, Ye W, Li X, Zhang J. Fatty liver decreases the risk of liver metastasis in patients with breast cancer: A two-center cohort study. Breast Cancer Research and Treatment. 2017;**166**(1):289-297

[26] Erler JT, Bennewith KL, Cox TR, Lang G, Bird D, Koong A, et al. Hypoxia-induced lysyl oxidase is a critical mediator of bone marrow cell recruitment to form the premetastatic niche. Cancer Cell. 2009;**15**(1):35-44

[27] Cox TR, Bird D, Baker AM, Barker HE, Ho MW, Lang G, et al. LOX-mediated collagen crosslinking is responsible for fibrosis-enhanced metastasis. Cancer Research. 2013;**73**(16):1721

[28] Kondo T, Okabayashi K, Hasegawa H, Tsuruta M, Shigeta K, Kitagawa Y. The impact of hepatic fibrosis on the incidence of liver metastasis from colorectal cancer. British Journal of Cancer. 2016;**115**(1):34

[29] Hussain SP, Harris CC. Inflammation and cancer: An ancient link with novel potentials. International Journal of Cancer. 2007;**121**(11):2373-2380

[30] Calzadilla Bertot L, Adams LA. The natural course of non-alcoholic fatty liver disease. International Journal of Molecular Sciences. 2016;**17**(5):774

[31] Sattar N, Forrest E, Preiss D. Non-alcoholic fatty liver disease. BMJ. 2014;**349**:g4596

[32] Arauz J, Ramos-Tovar E, Muriel P. Redox state and methods to evaluate oxidative stress in liver damage: From bench to bedside. Annals of Hepatology. 2016;**15**(2):160

[33] Augustin HG, Koh GY. Organotypic vasculature: From descriptive heterogeneity

to functional pathophysiology. Science. 2017;**357**(6353):eaal2379. DOI: 10.1126/science.aal2379

[34] Teng S, Li YE, Yang M, Qi R, Huang Y, Wang Q, et al. Tissue-specific transcription reprogramming promotes liver metastasis of colorectal cancer. Cell Research. 2019;**30**(1):34

[35] Wang C, Luo D. The metabolic adaptation mechanism of metastatic organotropism. Experimental Hematology & Oncology. 2021;**10**(1):30

[36] Orci LA, Lacotte S, Delaune V, Slits F, Oldani G, Lazarevic V, et al. Effects of the gut-liver axis on ischaemia-mediated hepatocellular carcinoma recurrence in the mouse liver. Journal of Hepatology. 2018;**68**(5):978-985

[37] Orci LA, Lacotte S, Oldani G, Morel P, Mentha G, Toso C. The role of hepatic ischemia-reperfusion injury and liver parenchymal quality on cancer recurrence. Digestive Diseases and Sciences. 2014;**59**(9):2058-2068

[38] Chen H, Lu D, Yang X, Hu Z, He C, Li H, et al. One shoot, two birds: Alleviating inflammation caused by ischemia/reperfusion injury to reduce the recurrence of hepatocellular carcinoma. Frontiers in Immunology. 2022;**13**:879552

[39] Zhang HF, Gao X, Wang X, Chen X, Huang Y, Wang L, et al. The mechanisms of renin-angiotensin system in hepatocellular carcinoma: From the perspective of liver fibrosis, HCC cell proliferation, metastasis and angiogenesis, and corresponding protection measures. Biomedicine & Pharmacotherapy. 2021;**141**:111868

[40] Wainwright P, Scorletti E, Byrne CD. Type 2 diabetes and hepatocellular carcinoma: Risk factors and pathogenesis. Current Diabetes Reports. 2017;**17**(4):20

[41] Singh MK, Das BK, Choudhary S, Gupta D, Patil UK. Diabetes and hepatocellular carcinoma: A pathophysiological link and pharmacological management. Biomedicine & Pharmacotherapy. 2018;**106**:991-1002

[42] Dellon ES, Shaheen NJ. Diabetes and hepatocellular carcinoma: Associations, biologic plausibility, and clinical implications. Gastroenterology. 2005;**129**(3):1132-1134

[43] Connolly GC, Safadjou S, Chen R, Nduaguba A, Dunne R, Khorana AA, et al. Diabetes mellitus is associated with the presence of metastatic spread at disease presentation in hepatocellular carcinoma. Cancer Investigation. 2012;**30**(10):698-702

[44] Yamashita T, Wang XW. Cancer stem cells in the development of liver cancer. Journal of Clinical Investigation. 2013;**123**(5):1911-1918

[45] Chen S, Cao Q, Wen W, Wang H. Targeted therapy for hepatocellular carcinoma: Challenges and opportunities. Cancer Letters. 2019;**28**(460):1-9

[46] Ohri N, Kaubisch A, Garg M, Guha C. Targeted therapy for hepatocellular carcinoma. Seminars in Radiation Oncology. 2016;**26**(4):338-343

[47] Ji J, Wang XW. New kids on the block: Diagnostic and prognostic microRNAs in hepatocellular carcinoma. Cancer Biology & Therapy. 2009;**8**(18):1686-1693

[48] Li Y, He X, Zhang X, Xu Y, Wu Y, Xu X. Immune-related microRNA signature for predicting prognosis

and the immune microenvironment in hepatocellular carcinoma. Life Sciences. 2021;**265**:118799

[49] Yang N, Ekanem NR, Sakyi CA, Ray SD. Hepatocellular carcinoma and microRNA: New perspectives on therapeutics and diagnostics. Advanced Drug Delivery Reviews. 2015;**81**:62-74

[50] Lou W, Chen J, Ding B, Chen D, Zheng H, Jiang D, et al. Identification of invasion-metastasis-associated microRNAs in hepatocellular carcinoma based on bioinformatic analysis and experimental validation. Journal of Translational Medicine. 2018;**16**(1):266

[51] Saito Y, Hibino S, Saito H. Alterations of epigenetics and microRNA in hepatocellular carcinoma. Hepatology Research. 2014;**44**(1):31-42

[52] Fornari F, Gramantieri L, Callegari E, Shankaraiah RC, Piscaglia F, Negrini M, et al. MicroRNAs in animal models of HCC. Cancers (Basel). 2019;**11**(12):1906

Chapter 4

Role of Biomarkers in Hepatocellular Carcinoma and Their Disease Progression

S.S. Haque, Ravi Bhushan Raman and Mehboobus Salam

Abstract

Hepatocellular carcinoma (HCC) is one of the third leading and common lethal cancers worldwide. Early detection of tumorigenesis of hepatocellular carcinoma is through ultrasonography, computerized tomography (CT) scans, and magnetic resonance imaging (MRI) scans; however, these methods are not up to the mark, so a search for an efficient biomarker for early diagnosis and treatment of hepatocarcinogenesis is important. Proteomic and genomic approaches aid to develop new promising biomarkers for the diagnosis of HCC at the early stages. These biomarkers not only help in prognosis but also provide better therapeutic intervention against HCC. Among the different biomarker candidates, liquid biopsy [including circulating tumor cells (CTCs) and circulating tumor DNA (ctDNA)] has recently emerged as a noninvasive detection technique for the characterization of circulating cells, providing a strong basis and early diagnosis for the individualized treatment of patients. This review provides the current understanding of HCC biomarkers that predict the risk of HCC recurrence.

Keywords: hepatocellular carcinoma, biomarkers, diagnosis, prognosis

1. Introduction

Hepatocellular carcinoma (HCC) is the fourth most common type of primary liver malignancy and is prevalent in almost most parts of the world [1]. Hepatitis B virus or hepatitis C virus is the most important contributing factor [2]. Liver biopsy is invasive but still the gold standard for determining the presence of the tumor. However, in some cases, preoperative biopsy of the tumor samples does not accurately predict microvascular invasion when compared with the final specimen examination after liver resection [3, 4]. Due to the risk of needle tract tumor seeding and other limitations, preoperative biopsy is not currently recommended for routine HCC evaluation. Biomarkers are biological indicator molecules of physiological and disease states. The detection of HCC in the blood is simple, noninvasive, reliable, and the best choice for screening of HCC. In the coming year, newly identified biomarkers will be more thoroughly evaluated for the diagnosis of HCC (**Figure 1**). In this review, some promising biomarkers are discussed.

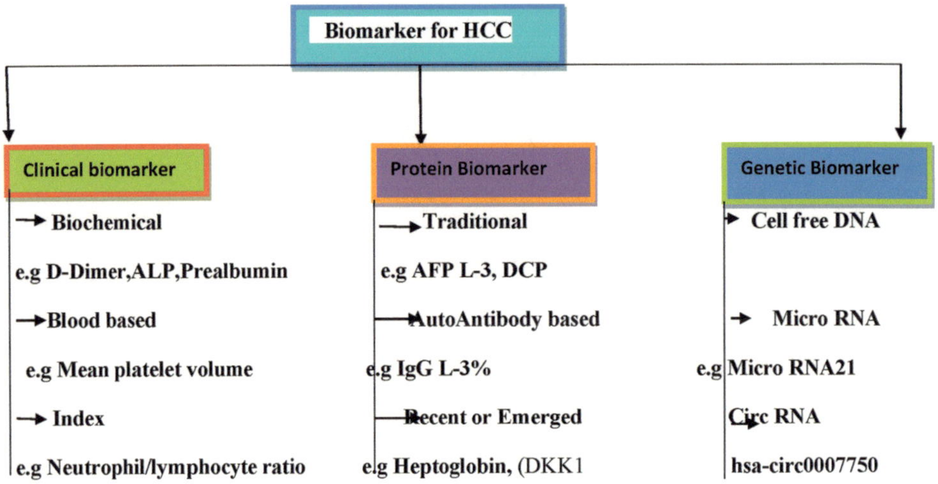

Figure 1.
Biomarker for HCC.

As a clinical biomarker, D-dimer is commonly used in HCC because portal vein thrombosis (PVT) is one of the important complications of HCC. D-dimer is the end product of fibrin degradation and is produced by fibrinogen, so D-dimer is a marker of endogenous fibrinolysis and its levels increase with fibrinolysis [5, 6]. Prealbumin (PA) or transthyretin is a homotetrameric protein that has been recently identified as a biomarker by the liver [7]. In contrast to albumin, prealbumin has a short biological half-life and reflects recent status [8]. Preoperative prealbumin level is useful for predicting long-term outcomes in patients undergoing liver resection for HCC.

The protein biomarker alpha-fetoprotein (AFP) is an important traditional diagnostic biomarker for hepatocellular carcinoma (HCC) for the past several decades. It is a 67-kDa glycoprotein that is produced by the liver in early fetal life when hepatocytes have not yet matured, and in HCC because of the dedifferentiation of hepatocytes to a more fetal pattern of gene expression. Serum AFP levels of more than 500 ng/ml are considered to have diagnostic significance; however, these values are reported only in a small percentage of patients with HCC. Many studies have reported that elevated serum AFP levels are correlated with increased risks of HCC in individuals infected with the hepatitis C virus (HCV) [9, 10]. In the practical aspects, the serum AFP concentrations do not correlate well with the prognostic values of HCC, such as the size of the tumor, stages, or disease progression, and ethnic variability may also be reported. Furthermore, in some cases of HCC, AFP elevations are not apparent at all and lack apparent discriminating power [11]. In HCC, the liver is damaged by one or more preexisting pathologic conditions, including cirrhosis and chronic hepatitis resulting from HBV or HCV infection [12], which also exhibited high serum AFP levels [13]. Three types of glycoforms of AFP have been identified so far, which are based on the difference in their binding affinities for Lens culinaris agglutinin (LCA). AFPL1 is a nonbinding fraction and AFP-L2 is a weakly binding fraction of total AFP. AFP-L3 is associated effectively with LCA [14], which is why it is a more specific biomarker for HCC. The AFP-L3 fraction has significantly increased the sensitivity for the early detection of HCC. However, AFP-based diagnostic approaches are still far from satisfactory results.

2. Serum autoantibodies

At an early stage of carcinogenesis, a small amount of tumor antigens can be produced by tumor cells that ultimately generate autoantibodies. These autoantibodies are stable in blood circulation and remain elevated for a long time [15]. IgG-L3% HCC-derived immunoglobulin G (IgG) and any type of unwanted glycosylations cause carcinogenesis. The fraction of Lens culinaris agglutinin-binding IgG (IgG-L3) among total serum IgG (IgG-L3%) increases with tumor load compared to healthy volunteers and asymptomatic HBV carriers.

3. Emerging serum protein biomarkers

Although traditional biomarkers have certain diagnostic values for HCC, none of them have been suitable in clinical practice, but there are emerging serum biomarkers. For example, aldo-keto reductase family 1 member B10 (AKR1B10) is a novel secretory protein that is associated with lung, breast, and colorectal cancers but induced in hepatocellular carcinoma (HCC), and this protein is located on chromosome 7q33 [16, 17] and is one of the important diagnostic and prognostic biomarkers for HCC [18–20]. AKR1B10 protein is an oncogenic protein that induces tumor development and progression by the removal of cytotoxic carbonyl compounds [21–23]. Dickkopf-1 (DKK1) is a 266-amino acid (35-kDa) secreted glycoprotein and antagonist of the Wnt/beta-catenin pathway signaling pathway discovered in 1998, which is expressed in a variety of human tumors. It is one of the impaired signaling pathways in hepatocellular carcinoma (HCC). Its function seems to be contradictory in the process of tumorigenesis, acting either as an oncogenic promoter of metastasis or as a tumor suppressor. In many tumors, high expression of *Dkk1* may promote tumor metastasis. However, *Dkk1* can inhibit tumor invasion and metastasis [24–26] and plays an important role in regulating human HCC cell migration, invasion, and tumor growth [27]. Therefore, novel genetic biomarkers for early diagnosis and detection are needed.

With the advent of cellular and molecular techniques for a better understanding of tumor biology, the role of biomarkers related to early detection has attracted a great deal of research interest resulting in the discovery and utilization of several novel markers in this disease. Liquid biopsy is one of the potential and noninvasive procedures that have attracted much attention to identify tumor markers in peripheral blood for diagnosis, monitoring, and prognosis of cancer, and overcoming tissue biopsy limitations. In this procedure, the sampling and analysis of biological samples, such as blood, urine, saliva, or stool, are done where nucleic acids originating from all or part of the body can be found including circulating tumor DNA (ctDNA) or RNA, exosomes, and circulating tumor cells (CTC). Most of the studies are carried out for mutations of ctDNA to detect minimal residual disease, as diagnostic markers or response to therapy. For the mapping of genetic alterations in ctDNA either next-generation sequencing (NGS) or digital PCR are used. Circulating tumoral cells and tumoral cell-free nucleic acids in peripheral blood could signal the presence of micrometastasis, and their utility has been explored in HCC diagnosis and prognosis.

Some other circulating RNAs have been explored, but none of them have been widely recognized as valuable markers of HCC recurrence, probably because none of them are specific for HCC [28]. In cancer biology, different types of circulating cellular elements have been identified as tumor markers [29, 30]. One of them is circulating tumor cells (CTC), which consist of obtaining a sample in a convenient and minimally invasive manner at multiple time points over the course of the disease.

4. Circulating tumor cells (CTCs)

Circulating tumor cells (CTCs) are defined as the primary solid tumor cells shed into blood, bone marrow or lymphatic vessels, or other healthy organs. These cells have a strong potential for distant metastasis, circulating through the bloodstream, and traveling to different tissues or organs of the body [31]. This type of tumor development process occurs at every stage. Australian doctor Thomas R. Ashworth was the first to discover CTCs in 1869 in the blood of a breast cancer patient [32]. CTCs are one of the useful markers for early diagnosis and monitoring of disease relapse. Their concentration is very low in blood, which limited the studies on CTC. Metastatic cells struggle to survive in the bloodstream and less than 0.01% of CTCs introduced into the circulation survive to produce metastases [33]. In recent years, with the advent of new technology, the separation and enrichment of CTCs have been greatly improved. In cancer, CTCs have received great attention in trying to estimate the future course in patients with breast cancer, colon cancer, and prostate cancer.

CTC analysis might provide personalized and effective strategies for clinicians and researchers because CTCs are sensitive biomarkers that enable early diagnosis, real-time monitoring, and molecular characterization to facilitate the implementation of precision medicine. In addition, the different study shows powerful evidence for the potential clinical value of the CTC assay [34]. However, numerous obstructions must be overcome before CTC analysis can be applied in the clinic. The CTC detection methods mentioned above have their own advantages and drawbacks. It is one of the important tasks to establish a highly sensitive and specific method that provides the full spectrum of CTCs. Therefore, the standardized method for CTC evaluation includes sample preparation, enrichment, and detection. In addition, lots of studies are single-center case-control research, with limited sample sizes. Validation is sometimes difficult or impossible to achieve. A multicenter prospective study with sufficient sample size and long follow-up is needed for CTC detection methodologies, the detection method must be uniform, and large samples can provide powerful validation for accurate analysis and standard evaluation of the final data. Although CTC detection is currently used in research, technological advancement will make it feasible in clinical practice in the near future.

5. Circulating tumor DNA (ctDNA)

Circulating tumor DNA (ctDNA) has attracted extensive attention for its wide application in cancer research, and it consists of mutant DNAs or tumor-derived fragmented DNA released into the circulation by tumor cells and constitute part of circulating cell-free DNA (cfDNA) in different types of cancer [35], cfDNA levels vary substantially from <0.01% to >60% of alleles in circulation [36, 37]. ctDNA carries the genetic information of the tumor, and it is highly specific and can detect at very low concentrations, making it suitable for early diagnosis, treatment, and monitoring of tumor progression. ctDNA is a liquid biopsy to profile the genome of a tumor more comprehensively than conventional sampling methods. Thus, it is an important tool to provide information for guiding targeted therapy [38], unveiling drug resistance [39], and monitoring treatment response [40]. Analysis of ctDNA helps in the efficient evaluation of disease status and early detection of recurrence, providing an average of 10–12 months' lead time for detection of metastatic recurrence compared to traditional modalities [41]. After resection, detectable ctDNA could identify cancer patients at high risk of recurrence, [42] while dynamic ctDNA changes can predict clinical relapse [43]. ctDNA provides information about specific tumor genes, such as DNA methylation, point mutations, copy number variations (CNVs), and chromosomal rearrangements. It also provides a unique opportunity for serially monitoring tumor genomes in a noninvasive, convenient, and accurate manner. Two different changes are monitored during the detection of ctDNA—quantitative changes and qualitative changes. The first detection method measures the quantity of ctDNA in circulation, and the second detects tumor-specific genetic aberrations. Many studies have carried out quantitative changes in cfDNA in the blood of HCC patients and show that elevated levels of cfDNA may represent an important complementary tool with potential clinical applications for detection, screening, treatment monitoring, and predicting metastatic potential [44–51].

Cell-free nucleic acids (cfNA) were first reported in human peripheral blood by Mandel and Metais in 1948 [52]. However, their studies did not recognize until 30 years later with the discovery of higher concentrations of cell-free DNA (cfDNA) in serum and plasma from cancer patients compared to healthy individuals. Currently, cfDNA is supposed to be released by normal cells at an average concentration of 30 ng/ml (0–100 ng/ml) into peripheral blood at the physiological level [53]. The concentration of cfDNA was accompanied by a decrease in DNase activity because cfDNA is degraded by peripheral blood deoxyribonuclease activity. Normal cells in peripheral circulation can also release cfDNA, and this reduces ctDNA concentrations [54]. cfDNA lysis occurs secondary to the clotting process of blood cells in collection tubes; thus, several studies have found significantly high cfDNA concentrations in serum than in plasma [55, 56]. Similarly, the blood specimen collected improperly or mechanical shearing leads to the destruction of the blood cells, causing the release of cfDNA into plasma [57]. Until recently, many researchers preferred plasma fraction over that in serum for cfDNA analysis [58]. Although DNA in the plasma is least contaminated with blood cells, the amount of DNA in plasma is more or less affected due to the time interval between analysis and blood collection [59].

A large number of hypermethylated genes, such as developing brain homeobox protein 2 (DBX2) [60], G-protein-coupled bile acid receptor (TGR5) [61], metallothionein 1M (MT1M), metallothionein 1G (MT1G) [62] and I the cyclin kinase inhibitor (NK4A) [63], were detected as cfDNA from HCC patients and were identified as biomarkers of vascular invasion. In the process of HCC diagnosis, high degree of methylation at multiple genes has been shown to play an important role. In addition, to improve the diagnostic efficiency, the combined detection of the methylation status of multiple genes may be effective [64].

The presence of cell-free DNA in plasma/serum has been used to reveal tumor-associated biomarkers, such as the increased plentiful of cell-free DNA (cfDNA) in cancer patients or the presence of epigenetic or specific genetic alterations, which have been discovered in numerous types of cancers, including HCC. Many studies have reported that the cfDNA is a source of HCC biomarkers in the diagnostic and prognosis of HCC in clinical settings also; HCC-specific biomarkers should be validated to determine their association with HCC recurrence. Finally, different micro (mi) RNA signatures in liver tissue have been associated with HCC [65, 66]. However, the necessity of obtaining liver tissue samples limits their application preoperatively, and circulating miRNAs are at present being explored. Several circulating miRNAs have been reported as important biomarkers for HCC diagnosis [67], prognosis, and vascular invasion [68, 69]. To date, there are no data about the association of miRNAs with HCC recurrence, and future studies are needed to explore the utility of these promising biomarkers.

6. Circulating microRNAs

Circulating microRNAs (miRNAs) were first proposed as potential cancer biomarkers in 2008 [70]. Blood miRNAs, which circulate in a highly stable, cell-free form, show promise as novel potential biomarkers for early detection of HCC. A number of evidence indicate that these noncoding nucleotide sequences are resistant to RNase degradation, repeated freeze-thaw cycles, boiling as well as acid/base treatment [71, 72]. The stability of circulating miRNAs has attracted attention from clinical researchers, who want to investigate their diagnostic utility for a wide range of diseases including HCC.

Under extreme conditions, their stability and their abundance in sera made circulating miRNAs as promising biomarkers for cancer pathologies [73, 74]. Serum miRNAs are not digested by ribonuclease because they are encapsulated in protein complexes or in membranous microvesicles that transport them in the circulatory system [75, 76]. The circulating miRNAs are stable when the samples are stored at −80°C [77]. Despite the valuable investigation of extracellular miRNAs, the use of miRNAs as biomarkers of cancer is still regarded as a "work in progress" and mostly confined to research programs [78]. Continuing technological advancements, however, like second-generation sequencing, as well as a perceptive of the pathobiological role of miRNAs, emphasize their future promise as clinical biomarkers [79].

7. Circular RNAs

Circular RNAs (circRNAs) are covalently closed, single-stranded, and stable RNA molecules [80] that have been evaluated for the diagnosis of various cancers. They contribute importantly to gastric cancer [81, 82], breast cancer [83], lung cancer [84, 85], pancreatic cancer [86], and HCC [87]. In a multicenter study, three circRNAs (hsa_circ_0000976, hsa_circ_0007750, and hsa_circ_0139897) were successfully validated in the plasma of the hepatitis B virus-related HCC patients, and their plasma levels positively correlated with HCC relapse, while after hepatectomy their levels decreased [87].

8. Conclusion

In the present scenario, no single or biomarker combination is predictable enough to diagnose a HCC lesion without confirmatory histological or radiological data. None of the new tumor markers excel the conventional ones in such a way that it has been widely endorsed in clinical practice. The liquid biopsy is one of the critical parts of precision medicine, and it is likely to be useful in the near future. However, future research should develop useful HCC biomarkers for monitoring treatment activity, detecting early resistance to treatment, and identifying patients who would more likely benefit from treatment.

We expect that identifying novel cost-effective and high-efficient biomarkers for the early diagnosis of HCC will be promising.

Author details

S.S. Haque[1*], Ravi Bhushan Raman[2] and Mehboobus Salam[3]

1 Department of Biochemistry, Indira Gandhi Institute of Medical Sciences, Patna, India

2 Department of Pathology (Hematology Section), Indira Gandhi Institute of Medical Sciences, Patna, India

3 Central Research Institute of Unani Medicine, Lucknow, India

*Address all correspondence to: sshaq2002@yahoo.co.in

References

[1] Njei B, Rotman Y, Ditah I, Lim JK. Emerging trends in hepatocellular carcinoma incidence and mortality. Hepatology. 2015;**61**:191-199

[2] Global Burden of Disease Liver Cancer Collaboration, Akinyemiju T, Abera S, Ahmed M, Alam N, Alemayohu MA, et al. Choi JAMA Oncology. 2017;**3**(12): 1683-1691. DOI: 10.1001/jamaoncol.2017

[3] Pawlik TM, Gleisner AL, Anders RA, Assumpcao L, Maley W, Choti MA. Preoperative assessment of hepatocellular carcinoma tumor grade using needle biopsy: Implications for transplant eligibility. Annals of Surgery. 2007;**245**:435-442

[4] Court CM, Harlander-Locke MP, Markovic D, French SW, Naini BV, Lu DS, et al. Determination of hepatocellular carcinoma grade by needle biopsy is unreliable for liver transplant candidate selection. Liver Transplantation. 2017;**23**:1123-1132

[5] Uccello M, Malaguarnera G, Pelligra EM, Biondi A, Basile F, Motta M. Lipoprotein(a) as a potential marker of residual liver function in hepatocellular carcinoma. Indian Journal of Medical and Paediatric Oncology. 2011;**32**(2):71-75

[6] Malaguarnera G, Gagliano C, Giordano M, et al. Homocysteine serum levels in diabetic patients with non proliferative, proliferative and without retinopathy. Biomed Research International. 2014;**2014**:1-4e191497

[7] Tripodi A. D-dimer testing in laboratory practice. Clinical Chemistry. 2011;**57**(9):1256-1262

[8] Kumada T et al. Predictive value of tumor markers for hepatocarcinogenesis in patients with hepatitis C virus. Journal of Gastroenterology. 2011;**46**:536-544

[9] Chen DS, Sung JL, Sheu JC. Serum α-fetoprotein in the early stage of human hepatocellular carcinoma. Gastroenterology. 1984;**86**(6):1404-1409

[10] Saffroy R et al. New perspectives and strategy research biomarkers for hepatocellular carcinoma. Clinical Chemistry and Laboratory Medicine. 2007;**45**:1169-1179

[11] Fattovich G et al. Hepatocellular carcinoma in cirrhosis: Incidence and risk factors. Gastroenterology. 2004;**127**(suppl. 1):S35-S50

[12] Lok AS, Lai CL. Alpha-fetoprotein monitoring in Chinese patients with chronic hepatitis B virus infection: Role in the early detection of hepatocellular carcinoma. Hepatology. 1989;**9**:110-115

[13] Li J, Han X, Yu X, Xu Z, Yang G, Liu B, et al. Clinical applications of liquid biopsy as prognostic and predictive biomarkers in hepatocellular carcinoma: Circulating tumor cells and circulating tumor DNA. Journal of Experimental and Clinical Cancer Research. 2018;**37**:213

[14] Schuler F, Dolken G. Detection and monitoring of minimal residual disease by quantitative real-time PCR. Clinica Chimica Acta. 2006;**363**:147-156.7

[15] Tan HT, Low J, Lim SG, Chung MC. Serum autoantibodies as biomarkers for early cancer detection. The FEBS Journal. 2009;**276**:6880-6904. DOI: 10.1111/j.1742-4658.2009.07396.x

[16] Wang NY, Wang C, Li W, Wang GJ, Cui GZ, He H, et al. Prognostic value of serum AFP, AFP-L3, and GP73 in monitoring short-term treatment

response and recurrence of hepatocellular carcinoma after radiofrequency ablation. Asian Pacific Journal of Cancer Prevention. 2014;**15**:1539-1544. DOI: 10.7314/APJCP.2014.15.4.1539

[17] Xia Y, Yan ZL, Xi T, Wang K, Li J, Shi LH, et al. A case control study of correlation between preoperative serum AFP and recurrence of hepatocellular carcinoma after curative hepatectomy. Hepato-Gastroenterology. 2012;**59**: 2248-2254. DOI: 10.5754/hge11978

[18] Bi X, Yan T, Zhao H, Zhao J, Li Z, Huang Z, et al. Correlation of alpha fetoprotein with the prognosis of hepatocellular carcinoma after hepatectomy in an ethnic Chinese population. Zhonghua Yi Xue Za Zhi. 2014;**94**:2645-2649. DOI: 10.3760/cma.j.issn.0376-2491.2014. 34.002

[19] Singal AG, Chan V, Getachew Y, Guerrero R, Reisch JS, Cuthbert JA. Predictors of liver transplant eligibility for patients with hepatocellular carcinoma in a safety net hospital. Digestive Diseases and Sciences. 2012;**57**:580-586. DOI: 10.1007/s10620-011-1904-7

[20] Eurich D, Boas-Knoop S, Morawietz L, Neuhaus R, Somasundaram R, Ruehl M, et al. Association of mannose-binding lectin-2 gene polymorphism with the development of hepatitis C-induced hepatocellular carcinoma. Liver International. 2011;**31**:1006-1012. DOI: 10.1111/j.1478-3231.2011.02522.x

[21] Zhong L, Liu Z, Yan R, Johnson S, Zhao Y, Fang X, et al. Aldo-Keto reductase family 1 B10 protein detoxifies dietary and lipid-derived alpha, beta-unsaturated carbonyls at physiological levels. Biochemical and Biophysical Research Communications. 2009;**387**(2):245-250. DOI: 10.1016/j.bbrc.2009.06.123

[22] Shen Y, Zhong L, Johnson S, Cao D. Human aldo-keto reductases 1B1 and 1B10: A comparative study on their enzyme activity toward electrophilic carbonyl compounds. Chemico-Biological Interactions. 2011;**191**(1-3):192-198. DOI: 10.1016/j.cbi.2011.02.004

[23] Yan R, Zu X, Ma J, Liu Z, Adeyanju M, Cao D. Aldo-keto reductase family 1 B10 gene silencing results in growth inhibition of colorectal cancer cells: Implication for cancer intervention. International Journal of Cancer. 2007;**121**(10):2301-2306. DOI: 10.1002/ijc.22933

[24] Liu C, Xiao GQ, Yan LN, Li B, Jiang L, Wen TF, et al. Value of alpha-fetoprotein in association with clinicopathological features of hepatocellular carcinoma. World Journal of Gastroenterology. 2013;**19**:1811-1819. DOI: 10.3748/wjg.v19.i11.1811

[25] Ilikhan SU, Bilici M, Sahin H, Akca AS, Can M, Oz II, et al. Assessment of the correlation between serum prolidase and alpha-fetoprotein levels in patients with hepatocellular carcinoma. World Journal of Gastroenterology. 2015;**21**:6999-7007. DOI: 10.3748/wjg.v21.i22.6999

[26] Abbasi A, Bhutto AR, Butt N, Munir SM. Corelation of serum alpha fetoprotein and tumor size in hepatocellular carcinoma. The Journal of the Pakistan Medical Association. 2012;**62**:33-36

[27] Tang H, Tang XY, Liu M, Li X. Targeting alpha-fetoprotein represses the proliferation of hepatoma cells via regulation of the cell cycle. Clinica Chimica Acta. 2008;**394**:81-88. DOI: 10.1016/j.cca.2008.04.012

[28] Dardaei L, Shahsavani R, Ghavamzadeh A, Behmanesh M, Aslankoohi E, Alimoghaddam K, et al. The detection of disseminated tumor cells in bone marrow and peripheral blood of gastric cancer patients by multimarker (CEA, CK20, TFF1 and MUC2) quantitative real-time PCR. Clinical Biochemistry. 2011;**44**:325-330

[29] Chaffer CL, Weinberg RA. A perspective on cancer cell metastasis. Science. 2011;**331**:1559-1564

[30] Ashworth T. A case of cancer in which cells similar to those in the tumours were seen in the blood after death. The Australasian Medical Journal. 1869;**14**:146-149

[31] Ma J, Yan R, Zu X, Cheng JM, Rao K, Liao DF, et al. Aldo-keto reductase family 1 B10 affects fatty acid synthesis by regulating the stability of acetylCoA carboxylase-alpha in breast cancer cells. Journal of Biological Chemistry. 2008;**283**:3418-3423. DOI: 10.1074/jbc.M707650200

[32] Ashworth TR. A case of cancer in which cells similar to those in the tumours were seen in the blood after death. The Australasian Medical Journal. 1869;**14**:146-147

[33] Tremblay PL, Huot J, Auger FA. Mechanisms by which E-selectin regulates diapedesis of colon cancer cells under flow conditions. Cancer Research. 2008;**68**(13):5167-5176. DOI: 10.1158/0008-5472.CAN-08-1229

[34] Alunni-Fabbroni M, Sandri MT. Circulating tumour cells in clinical practice: Methods of detection and possible characterization. Methods. 2010;**50**:289-297

[35] Han C, Gao L, Bai H, Dou X. Identification of a role for serum aldoketo reductase family 1 member B10 in early detection of hepatocellular carcinoma. Oncology Letters. 2018;**16**:7123-7130. DOI: 10.3892/ol.2018.9547

[36] Zhu R, Xiao J, Luo D, Dong M, Sun T, Jin J. Serum AKR1B10 predicts the risk of hepatocellular carcinoma—A retrospective single-center study. Gastroenterología y Hepatología. 2019;**42**:614-621. DOI: 10.1016/j.gastrohep.2019.06.007

[37] Ye X, Li C, Zu X, Lin M, Liu Q, Liu J, et al. A large-scale multicenter study validates AKR1B10 as a new prevalent serum marker for detection of hepatocellular carcinoma. Hepatology. 2019;**69**:2489-2501. DOI: 10.1002/hep.30519

[38] Sato N, Yamabuki T, Takano A, Koinuma J, Aragaki M, Masuda K, et al. Wnt inhibitor Dickkopf-1 as a target for passive cancer immunotherapy. Cancer Research. 2010;**70**:5326-5336. DOI: 10.1158/0008-5472.CAN-09-3879

[39] Rachner TD, Thiele S, Gobel A, Browne A, Fuessel S, Erdmann K, et al. High serum levels of Dickkopf-1 are associated with a poor prognosis in prostate cancer patients. BMC Cancer. 2014;**14**:649. DOI: 10.1186/1471-2407-14-649

[40] Peng YH, Xu YW, Guo H, Huang LS, Tan HZ, Hong CQ, et al. Combined detection of serum Dickkopf-1 and its autoantibodies to diagnose esophageal squamous cell carcinoma. Cancer Medicine. 2016;**5**:1388-1396. DOI: 10.1002/cam4.702

[41] Tung EK, Mak CK, Fatima S, Lo RC, Zhao H, Zhang C, et al. Clinicopathological and prognostic significance of serum and tissue Dickkopf-1 levels in human hepatocellular carcinoma. Liver

International. 2011;**31**:1494-1504. DOI: 10.1111/j.1478-3231.2011.02597.x

[42] Yin CQ, Yuan CH, Qu Z, Guan Q, Chen H, Wang FB. Liquid biopsy of hepatocellular carcinoma: Circulating tumor-derived biomarkers. Disease Markers. 2016;**2016**:1427849

[43] Miller MC, Doyle GV, Terstappen LW. Significance of circulating tumor cells detected by the cell search system in patients with metastatic breast colorectal and prostate cancer. Journal of Oncology. 2010;**2010**:617421

[44] Sun C, Liao W, Deng Z, Li E, Feng Q, Lei J, et al. The diagnostic value of assays for circulating tumor cells in hepatocellular carcinoma: A meta-analysis. Medicine. 2017;**96**(29):e7513. DOI: 10.1097/MD.0000000000007513

[45] Bettegowda C, Sausen M, Leary RJ, Kinde I, Wang Y, Agrawal N, et al. Detection of circulating tumor DNA in early- and late-stage human malignancies. Science Translational Medicine. 2014;**6**:224ra224

[46] Leung F, Kulasingam V, Diamandis EP, Hoon DS, Kinzler K, Pantel K, et al. Circulating tumor DNA as a cancer biomarker: Fact or fiction? Clinical Chemistry. 2016;**62**:1054-1060. DOI: 10.1373/clinchem.2016.260331

[47] Wong SQ, Raleigh JM, Callahan J, Vergara IA, Ftouni S, Hatzimihalis A, et al. Circulating tumor DNA analysis and functional imaging provide complementary approaches for comprehensive disease monitoring in metastatic melanoma. JCO Precision Oncology. 2017;**1**:1-14. DOI: 10.1200/PO.16.00009

[48] Luke JJ, Oxnard GR, Paweletz CP, Camidge DR, Heymach JV, Solit DB, et al. Cell free DNAWG. Realizing the potential of plasma genotyping in an age of genotype-directed therapies. Journal of the National Cancer Institute. 2014;**106**(8):dju214

[49] Murtaza M, Dawson SJ, Tsui DW, Gale D, Forshew T, Piskorz AM, et al. Non-invasive analysis of acquired resistance to cancer therapy by sequencing of plasma DNA. Nature. 2013;**497**:108-112

[50] Montagut C, Siravegna G, Bardelli A. Liquid biopsies to evaluate early therapeutic response in colorectal cancer. Annals of Oncology. 2015;**26**:1525-1527

[51] Reinert T, Scholer LV, Thomsen R, Tobiasen H, Vang S, Nordentoft I, et al. Analysis of circulating tumour DNA to monitor disease burden following colorectal cancer surgery. Gut. 2016;**65**:625-634

[52] Sausen M, Phallen J, Adleff V, Jones S, Leary RJ, Barrett MT, et al. Clinical implications of genomic alterations in the tumour and circulation of pancreatic cancer patients. Nature Communications. 2015;**6**:7686. DOI: 10.1038/ncomms8686

[53] Garcia-Murillas I, Schiavon G, Weigelt B, Ng C, Hrebien S, Cutts RJ, et al. Mutation tracking in circulating tumor DNA predicts relapse in early breast cancer. Science Translational Medicine. 2015;**7**:302ra133

[54] Mandel P, Métais P. Les acides nucleiques du plasma sanguin chez l'homme. Comptes Rendus de l'Académie des Sciences de Paris. 1948;**142**:241-243

[55] Sorenson GD, Pribish DM, Valone FH, Memoli VA, Bzik DJ, Yao S-L. Soluble normal and mutated DNA sequences from single-copy genes in human blood. Cancer Epidemiology, Biomarkers and Prevention. 1994;**3**(1): 67-71

[56] Fleischhacker M, Schmidt B. Circulating nucleic acids (CNAs) and cancer—A survey. Biochimica et Biophysica Acta. 2007;**1775**(1):181-232

[57] Ren N, Qin LX, Tu H, Liu YK, Zhang BH, Tang ZY. The prognostic value of circulating plasma DNA level and its allelic imbalance on chromosome 8p in patients with hepatocellular carcinoma. Journal of Cancer Research and Clinical Oncology. 2006;**132**(6):399-407

[58] Iizuka N, Sakaida I, Moribe T, Fujita N, Miura T, Stark M, et al. Elevated levels of circulating cell-free DNA in the blood of patients with hepatitis C virus-associated hepatocellular carcinoma. Anticancer Research. 2006;**26**(6C):4713-4719

[59] Yang YJ, Chen H, Huang P, Li CH, Dong ZH, Hou YL. Quantification of plasma hTERT DNA in hepatocellular carcinoma patients by quantitative fluorescent polymerase chain reaction. Clinical and Investigative Medicine. 2011;**34**(4):E238

[60] Piciocchi M, Cardin R, Vitale A, Vanin V, Giacomin A, Pozzan C, et al. Circulating free DNA in the progression of liver damage to hepatocellular carcinoma. Hepatology International. 2013;**7**(4):1050-1057

[61] Huang A, Zhang X, Zhou SL, Cao Y, Huang XW, Fan J, et al. Plasma circulating cell-free DNA integrity as a promising biomarker for diagnosis and surveillance in patients with hepatocellular carcinoma. Journal of Cancer. 2016;**7**(13):1798-1803

[62] Yan L, Chen Y, Zhou J, Zhao H, Zhang H, Wang G. Diagnostic value of circulating cell-free DNA levels for hepatocellular carcinoma. International Journal of Infectious Diseases. 2017;**67**:92-97

[63] Bettegowda C, Sausen M, Leary RJ, Kinde I, Wang Y, Agrawal N, et al. Detection of circulating tumor DNA in early and late-stage human malignancies. Science Translational Medicine. 2014;**6**(224):224ra224

[64] Diehl F, Schmidt K, Choti MA, Romans K, Goodman S, Li M, et al. Circulating mutant DNA to assess tumor dynamics. Nature Medicine. 2008;**14**(9):985-990

[65] Tamkovich SN, Cherepanova AV, Kolesnikova EV, Rykova EY, Pyshnyi DV, Vlassov VV, et al. Circulating DNA and DNase activity in human blood. Annals of the New York Academy of Sciences. 2006;**1075**:191-196

[66] Lee TH, Montalvo L, Chrebtow V, Busch MP. Quantitation of genomic DNA in plasma and serum samples: Higher concentrations of genomic DNA found in serum than in plasma. Transfusion. 2001;**41**(2):276-282

[67] Jung M, Klotzek S, Lewandowski M, Fleischhacker M, Jung K. Changes in concentration of DNA in serum and plasma during storage of blood samples. Clinical Chemistry. 2003;**49** (6 Pt 1):1028-1029

[68] Volik S, Alcaide M, Morin RD, Collins C. Cell-free DNA (cfDNA): Clinical significance and utility in cancer shaped by emerging technologies. Molecular Cancer Research. 2016;**14**(10): 898-908

[69] Vallee A, Marcq M, Bizieux A, Kouri CE, Lacroix H, Bennouna J, et al. Plasma is a better source of tumor-derived circulating cell-free DNA than serum for the detection of EGFR alterations in lung tumor patients. Lung Cancer. 2013;**82**(2):373-374

[70] van Dessel LF, Beije N, Helmijr JC, Vitale SR, Kraan J, Look MP, et al.

Application of circulating tumor DNA in prospective clinical oncology trials—Standardization of preanalytical conditions. Molecular Oncology. 2017;**11**(3):295-304

[71] Liese J, Peveling-Oberhag J, Doering C, Schnitzbauer AA, Herrmann E, Zangos S, et al. A possible role of microRNAs as predictive markers for the recurrence of hepatocellular carcinoma after liver transplantation. Transplant International. 2016;**29**: 369-380

[72] Han ZB, Zhong L, Teng MJ, Fan JW, Tang HM, Wu JY, et al. Identification of recurrence-related microRNAs in hepatocellular carcinoma following liver transplantation. Molecular Oncology. 2012;**6**:445-457

[73] Bharali D, Jebur HB, Baishya D, Kumar S, Sarma MP, Masroor M, et al. Expression analysis of serum microRNA-34a and microRNA-183 in hepatocellular carcinoma. Asian Pacific Journal of Cancer Prevention. 2018;**19**:2561-2568

[74] Cho HJ, Kim SS, Nam JS, Kim JK, Lee JH, Kim B, et al. Low levels of circulating microRNA-26a/29a as poor prognostic markers in patients with hepatocellular carcinoma who underwent curative treatment. Clinics and Research in Hepatology and Gastroenterology. 2017;**41**:181-189

[75] Zhang J, Lin H, Wang XY, Zhang DQ, Chen JX, Zhuang Y, et al. Predictive value of microRNA-143 in evaluating the prognosis of patients with hepatocellular carcinoma. Cancer Biomarkers. 2017;**19**: 257-262

[76] Zhang P, Wen X, Gu F, Deng X, Li J, Dong J, et al. Methylation profiling of serum DNA from hepatocellular carcinoma patients using an Infinium human methylation 450 BeadChip. Hepatology International. 2013;7(3):893-900

[77] Chen LL. The biogenesis and emerging roles of circular RNAs. Nature Reviews. Molecular Cell Biology. 2016;**17**:205-211. DOI: 10.1038/nrm.2015.32

[78] Sun H, Tang W, Rong D, Jin H, Fu K, Zhang W, et al. Hsa_circ_0000520, a potential new circular RNA biomarker, is involved in gastric carcinoma. Cancer Biomarkers. 2018;**21**:299-306. DOI: 10.3233/CBM-170379

[79] Li P, Chen S, Chen H, Mo X, Li T, Shao Y, et al. Using circular RNA as a novel type of biomarker in the screening of gastric cancer. Clinica Chimica Acta. 2015;**444**:132-136. DOI: 10.1016/j.cca.2015.02.018

[80] Li T, Shao Y, Fu L, Xie Y, Zhu L, Sun W, et al. Plasma circular RNA profiling of patients with gastric cancer and their droplet digital RT-PCR detection. Journal of Molecular Medicine. 2018;**96**:85-96. DOI: 10.1007/s00109-017-1600-y

[81] Yin WB, Yan MG, Fang X, Guo JJ, Xiong W, Zhang RP. Circulating circular RNA hsa_circ_0001785 acts as a diagnostic biomarker for breast cancer detection. Clinica Chimica Acta. 2018;**487**:363-368. DOI: 10.1016/j.cca.2017.10.011

[82] Zhu X, Wang X, Wei S, Chen Y, Chen Y, Fan X, et al. hsa_circ_0013958: A circular RNA and potential novel biomarker for lung adenocarcinoma. FEBS Journal. 2017;**284**:2170-2182. DOI: 10.1111/febs.14132

[83] Hang D, Zhou J, Qin N, Zhou W, Ma H, Jin G, et al. A novel plasma circular RNA circFARSA is a potential biomarker for non-small cell lung cancer. Cancer Medicine. 2018;7:2783-2791. DOI: 10.1002/cam4.1514

[84] Yang F, Liu DY, Guo JT, Ge N, Zhu P, Liu X, et al. Circular RNA circLDLRAD3 as a biomarker in diagnosis of pancreatic cancer. World Journal of Gastroenterology. 2017;**23**:8345-8354. DOI: 10.3748/wjg.v23.i47.8345

[85] Zhang X, Xu Y, Qian Z, Zheng W, Wu Q, Chen Y, et al. circRNA_104075 stimulates YAP-dependent tumorigenesis through the regulation of HNF4a and may serve as a diagnostic marker in hepatocellular carcinoma. Cell Death and Disease. 2018;**9**:1091. DOI: 10.1038/s41419-018-1132-6

[86] Li Z, Zhou Y, Yang G, He S, Qiu X, Zhang L, et al. Using circular RNA SMARCA5 as a potential novel biomarker for hepatocellular carcinoma. Clinica Chimica Acta. 2019;**492**:37-44. DOI: 10.1016/j.cca.2019.02.001

[87] Yu J, Ding WB, Wang MC, Guo XG, Xu J, Xu QG, et al. Plasma circular RNA panel to diagnose hepatitis B virus-related hepatocellular carcinoma: A large-scale, multicenter study. International Journal of Cancer. 2019;**146**:1754-1763. DOI: 10.1002/ijc.32647

Chapter 5

miRNAs in Liver Cancer

Alisa Petkevich, Aleksandr Abramov and Vadim Pospelov

Abstract

miRNAs are small noncoding RNAs, which are involved in epigenetic regulation of gene expression. Hepatocellular carcinoma (HCC), although not being at the top of most widespread cancers, nevertheless, remains among cancers with the most lethal cases. The chapter is dedicated to the epigenetic aspect of HCC development, namely the role of miRNA in this process. Being small and noncoding RNAs, they have a huge and significant function in gene regulation. This chapter will briefly cover following questions: miRNA biogenesis and function, metabolic and signaling pathways disrupted in HCC with a significant miRNA involvement, and main miRNAs contributing to HCC development and their targets.

Keywords: miRNA, hepatocellular carcinoma, target gene, gene expression, miRNA expression, diagnostic marker

1. Introduction

miRNAs are small noncoding RNAs ~20–25 nt long, which are involved in epigenetic regulation of gene expression. miRNAs were firstly discovered in 1993, when research groups led by Victor Ambros and Gary Ruvkun published two side-by-side papers in the journal Cell, describing the regulatory effects of tiny RNA discovered in Caenorhabditis elegans. Years later the term "microRNA" (miRNA, miR) was introduced [1]. Nowadays, more than 2600 miRNAs have been predicted to be encoded by the human genome, with the ability to modulate more than 15,000 genes [2]. Being small and noncoding RNAs, they have a huge and significant function in gene regulation and cancer development. Liver cancer, although not being at the top of most common cancers, remains among cancers with high mortality. Hepatocellular carcinoma (HCC) accounts for approximately 80% of all liver cancers and is a main cause of cancer mortality [3]. Hereinafter, when using the term liver cancer, it is meant to indicate hepatocellular carcinoma. The most obvious and significant reason for this high mortality rate in HCC patients is the late diagnosis of HCC. Against this background, every aspect of molecular pathogenesis becomes a valuable detail, which may aid in understanding HCC development. Some of the main miRNAs involved in the development of liver cancer will be discussed further. Changes in their expression levels were detected in comparable conditions: mostly in human liver tissue samples or human blood samples (plasma or serum) by qRT-PCR.

2. miRNA biogenesis and regulation

Despite the simple structure of a mature miRNA molecule—single-stranded RNA molecule of 20–25 nt—its biogenesis, like almost any process relating to nucleic acids, is multistage and multifactorial: It takes place both in the nucleus and in the cell cytoplasm, involves protein complexes for processing (miRNA maturation), may be performed *via* canonical and non-canonical pathways, and includes following transformations: primary miRNA (pri-miRNA), preliminary miRNA (pre-miRNA), miRNA duplex, and mature miRNA. Both canonical and non-canonical processing start in the nucleus.

miRNA processing may occur post- or co-transcriptionally [4]. miRNA biogenesis starts in the nucleus and requires RNA polymerase II/III; Drosha (an RNase III-like enzyme) with its cofactor, the RNA binding protein DGCR8 (DiGeorge Syndrome Critical Region 8), forms a microprocessor complex and functions in the nucleus, an exportin (frequently Exportin5 in the canonical pathway and Exportin1 in the non-canonical pathway) functioning as the transporter to the cytoplasm. Dicer, another RNase III-like endonuclease, RISC (RNA-induced silencing complex) functioning in the cytoplasm with Argonaute (AGO) as a core component. miRNA biogenesis starts with the processing of RNA polymerase II/III and forming pri-miRNAs, which are 5′ capped and 3′ polyadenylated, approximately several kilobases [5, 6]. In the canonical pathway, pri-miRNAs then are processed in the microprocessor complex of Drosha and DGCR8. The resulting ~70 nucleotide RNAs with 2 nt 3′ overhang are known as precursor (pre-) miRNAs, which fold into mini-helical structures [7]. Pre-miRNAs are transported from the nucleus to the cytoplasm with Exportin 5/RanGTP complex, where they undergo processing with Dicer, which recognizes the pre-miRNA hairpin and cuts it at the loop end, resulting in the removal of the terminal loop and creating a ~22 nt RNA duplex [8]. The final step of the miRNA biogenesis is processing the duplex miRNA into mature single-stranded miRNA by loading it onto an Argonaute (Ago) protein, which is the core protein in this final effector complex—RNA-induced silencing complex (RISC). The mature miRNA may be derived from both the 5' and 3' arms of the precursor duplex and are called the miRNA-5p and -3p, respectively [9].

As for regulation of miRNA expression with some miRNAs having their own promotors and some being regulated by other gene promotors, besides methylation, different endogenous factors, and hypoxia, different transcription factors (TF) also participate in miRNAs expression regulation and this is a double-edged process: TFs influence miRNA expression and miRNAs may repress TF expression [7, 10]. miRNA, TFs, and target genes form a complex relationship known as feedback loops (FBLs) and feed-forward loops (FFLs) [11]. Typically, FBLs occur when a TF activates or represses a miRNA, which in turn represses the TF; the miRNA and TF each regulate independent sets of TGs. FFLs are those where a regulator, such as a TF, controls the expression of a specific TG both directly, through promoting or enhancing its transcription, and indirectly, through another regulator, such as an miRNA that also regulates the TG [12].

mRNA and miRNA interaction implies binding of the last to the 3′ untranslated region (3′ UTR) of mRNA through base-pairing of the seed region of target mRNA, mainly at position 2–7 from the 5′ end of the miRNA; beyond the seed region, the binding between the whole mature miRNA sequence and the target mRNA is not perfectly complementary [13]. However, the interaction of miRNAs with other regions, including the 5′ UTR, coding sequence, and gene promoters, has also been reported.

In general, there is no direct correlation between miRNA and target mRNA expression levels. Multiple miRNAs can regulate a single gene/mRNA, and some miRNAs can target many mRNAs (up to more than 100 mRNAs) and from 1 to 2% of human transcripts interact with nine or more miRNAs, thus displaying sponge-like activity [14]. Furthermore, miRNAs have been shown to activate gene expression under certain conditions [5]. Along with mRNAs differing in their miRNA-binding capacity, binding activity of some highly expressed miRNAs may be weakened by either a high target-to-miRNA ratio or the relocation of this miRNA to the nucleus. Some miRNAs might be expressed at relatively low levels and interact with many mRNAs and, oppositely, some miRNAs might be expressed at a very high level and interact with only a few mRNAs [15].

Considering all of the above, it makes identifying the specific miRNA-target gene or transcription factor-target gene interactions difficult, and possibly unwarranted [12].

3. miRNA in liver functions

Apparently, miRNAs are involved in all processes underlying normal liver functioning, so main pathologic processes, such as nonalcoholic fatty liver disease (NAFLD), fibrosis at the background of various diseases, and cancer are associated with significant changes in miRNA expression profiles, although these changes are not always associated with target mRNA expression changes and the mechanism of miRNA participation in these processes is not clear. A significant role of some miRNAs was shown for main liver functions such as lipid metabolism and all the steps of glucose metabolism, including lipogenesis.

3.1 miRNAs and the regulation of lipid metabolism

Pivotal role of miR-34a in PPARα (the peroxisome proliferator-activated receptor alpha) pathway, which is a direct target of miR-34a and a master regulator of lipid metabolism, was shown in cultured cells transfected with miR-34a inhibitor and simultaneously consequences of miR-34a inhibition were shown in C57BL/6 mice injected with the miR-34a inhibitor [16]. The upregulation of miR-34a resulted in the downregulation of hepatic PPARα and SIRT1 (silent mating type information regulation 2 homolog 1), silencing miR-34a led to an initially increased expression of PPARα, SIRT1, and PPARα's downstream genes, and activation of the central metabolic sensor AMPK was also increased. In the mouse model, the miR-34a inhibitor suppressed lipid accumulation and improved the degree of steatosis, which is assumed to be regular as far as its level was significantly upregulated in liver tissues of high-fat diet-fed mice [17].

miR-122 is among those playing a crucial role in lipid metabolism in the liver: miR-122 expression in mice liver was increased by free fatty acids (FFAs) *via* activating the retinoic acid-related orphan receptor-alpha, inducing secretion of miR-122 to blood, entering muscle and adipose tissues of mice, reducing mRNA levels of genes involved in triglyceride synthesis, mainly, Agpat1 and Dgat1. It also led to the attenuated triglyceride synthesis and elevated β-oxidation pathway [18]. Before it was shown that cholesterol biosynthesis genes would be affected by miR-122, plasma cholesterol levels were reduced in antagomir-122-treated mice, thus illustrating attenuation of the cholesterol biosynthesis when silencing hepatic miR-122 [19]. There are another data, also proving the meaning of miR-122 in lipid metabolism, its inhibition in normal mice resulted in reduced plasma cholesterol levels, increased hepatic fatty-acid oxidation, and a decrease in hepatic fatty-acid and cholesterol synthesis rates. Simultaneously, miR-122 inhibition in a diet-induced obesity mouse model also resulted in decreased plasma cholesterol levels and a significant improvement in liver steatosis, accompanied by reductions in several lipogenic genes [20]. An increase in miR-122 expression in obese subjects may appear to be the compensated mechanism to maintain lipid metabolism. Besides miRNAs, hepatic lipid accumulation recruits inflammatory response, impairing some signaling pathways involved in lipid metabolism, including the AMPK signaling pathway, the role of miR-122 in energy metabolism in the liver, skeletal muscle, and adipose tissues requires more evidence to evaluate [21].

Among other miRNAs, possibly acting as modulators of lipid and cholesterol levels in the maintenance of cholesterol and fatty acid metabolism, are miR-33, miR-103, miR-104, and miR-307 [22, 23]. Obviously, some miRNAs may be involved in both lipid and glucose metabolisms, as far as one miRNA may have multiple mRNA targets. One of these miRNAs is miR-33a and miR-33b, intronic miRNAs located within the sterol regulatory element-binding protein (SREBP) genes, working in concert with its host gene to ensure a fine-tuned regulation of lipid and glucose homeostasis. miR33b also cooperates with SREBP1, having an impact on key regulatory enzymes of hepatic gluconeogenesis glucose metabolism—phosphoenolpyruvate carboxykinase (PCK1) and glucose-6-phosphatase (G6PC). Overexpression of miR-33b in human hepatic cells leads to a significant reduction of glucose production *via* inhibition of PCK1 and G6PC expression [24].

miR-206 was shown as a potent lipid and glucose production inhibitor by simultaneously facilitating insulin signaling and impairing hepatic lipogenesis due to promoting phosphorylation of INSR (insulin receptor) and impaired hepatic lipogenesis by inhibiting Srebp1 (sterol regulatory element-binding transcription factor 1) transcription and inhibition of PTPN1 (protein tyrosine phosphatase, non-receptor type 1) *via* interaction with its 3′ untranslated region and following degradation. miR-206 reduced lipid and glucose production in human hepatocytes and livers of dietary obese mice [25].

3.2 miRNAs and insulin signaling

miR-103 and miR-107 were the first two miRNAs shown to regulate insulin sensitivity in liver and adipose tissue in mice: Their overexpression in these mouse models led to downregulation of caveolin-1 expression, a component of caveolae lipid raft required for insulin receptor signaling. miR-802 was also shown to be involved in the regulation of insulin sensitivity and glucose transport: elevated miR-802 decreased expression of HNF1β while increasing expression of the insulin suppressors, SOCS1 and SOCS3. Increased expression of both SOCS1 and SOCS2, in turn, desensitizes insulin signaling, resulting in increased hepatic glucose production in these mouse models [26]. It is worth noting that miR-23a was first reported as a regulator of gluconeogenesis through direct binding at the 3’-UTRs of both G6Pase and PGC-1α mRNAs, and later its expression was found to be elevated in hepatocytes of hepatocellular carcinoma mice where gluconeogenesis is attenuated [27].

3.3 Circular RNAs

In general, when discussing miRNA functions and interactions, it should be noted, besides its elusive relations with mRNA, that they are not limited to mRNA and involve other RNAs as well, that may influence its activity and function, for example, circRNAs have been validated as microRNA (miRNA) sponges, which have complementary sequences binding to their target miRNAs, thereby inhibiting the function of those miRNAs and abolishing the inhibition of target gene expression [27]. Circ-0000092 with such miRNA sponging activity and miR-338-3p as a target miRNA was shown to be elevated in HCC tissue (40 patients, RT-qPCR, GAPDH) and cell lines, while miR-338-3p was shown to be decreased (40 patients, RT-qPCR, U6 as an internal control) [28]. Simultaneously, miRNA-338-3p target, HN1, shown to be overexpressed by Liu et al. in liver cancer and known to be involved in metastasis and invasion development in breast and prostate cancer partly due to negative impact on the b-catenin/E-cadherin interaction, was shown to be elevated along with circ-0000092 [29]. These data along with the effects of delivery of a series of mimic, inhibitor, or siRNA plasmids into HCC cells on cell proliferation, migration, invasion, and angiogenesis *in vitro* may allow to assume that circ-0000092, absorbing miRNA-338-3p and positively influencing HN1 expression, and promote cancer cell proliferation and invasion. A possible mechanism for maintaining CSC (cancer stem cell) self-renewal with HN1 involvement is enhancing of oncogenic factor MYC, and the LEPR–STAT3 pathway [29]. Another circRNA with specific sponging activity for miRNA-338-3p is circMAT2Bm, which also negatively influences miRNA-338-3p and, as a result, positively one of its targets—PKM2, which encodes one of the key enzymes in the process of glycolysis [30]. CircASAP1 in liver cancer acts as a competing endogenous RNA for miRNA-326 and miRNA-532-5p, which play a tumor suppressor role in liver cancer, regulating MAPK1 and CSF1. CircUHRF1, which is predominantly secreted into plasma in exosomes by HCC cells, inhibits the activity of miRNA-449, upregulating the expression of TIM3 and inhibiting NK cell function. The expression of circUHRF1 is higher in HCC tissues than in corresponding adjacent nontumor tissues [31]. There are other circRNAs, whose expression level is decreased in HCC tissues compared with noncancerous tissues, and that were shown to have miRNAs among their targets, such as circTRIM33-12 and miRNA-191, circHIAT1 and miRNA-3171, circLARP4 and miRNA-761, and circMTO1 and miRNA9. Decreased expression of these circRNAs in HCC resulted in elevated expression level of the corresponding miRNAs and sustaining of proliferation, invasion, and metastasis of cancer cells [31].

4. miRNA expression patterns in HCC

It is evident that most of the processes taking place in the liver in normal condition require different miRNAs and assumably healthy hepatocyte should have its "normal" miRNA profile with wide ranges, which make it possible to suggest—there are strong pieces of evidence that will be discussed further—those different pathologic processes, forming the diseases, are accompanied with different changes in miRNA expression levels. With regard to hepatocellular carcinoma, it could be speculated that in the very initial stages, particularly at preclinical stages when it is favorable for cancer background but still no clinical manifestation of cancer, liver cancer may have different miRNA expression profiles within the same cancer type. Further will be discussed the liver cancer development and partly the background of viral hepatitis B, viral hepatitis C, nonalcoholic fatty liver disease (NAFLD), and alcohol-related liver disease (ARLD).

miRNAs along with other nucleic acids have a significant impact on cancer development, where they may have both the role of cancer promotion and cancer suppression; therefore, miRNAs with increased expression in tumors are thought to function as oncogenes and are termed as oncomirs. On the contrary, miRNAs with decreased expression in cancer cells are considered tumor suppressor genes, presumably preventing tumor development by negatively inhibiting oncogenes and/or genes that control cell differentiation or apoptosis [32]. miRNAs are known to be involved in most signaling pathways, and in the liver cancer development, the same signaling pathways are involved, like in most other cancer types, such as TGF-β, Wnt/B-catenin, Hh, Notch, EGF, HGF, VEFG, JAK/STAT, Hippo, and HIF, which lead to uncontrolled cell division and metastasis [32].

Main miRNAs, involved in TGF-β regulation, are miR-200, miR-21, miR-211, miR-17/92, miR-106b/25, and miR-182 [33]. miR-200 and miR-21 are one of the main players among noncoding RNAs in interaction with TGF-β signaling in the process of EMT. miR-200 forming a double-negative feedback loop with ZEB factors (zinc finger E-box-binding homeobox) plays a significant role in EMT (epithelial-mesenchymal transition): miR-200 is downregulated because of reversible DNA methylation of the miR-200 loci as a result of prolonged autocrine TGF-β signaling, driving a sustained ZEB expression, and thus maintaining a stable mesenchymal phenotype. miR-200 is known to interact with both ZEB factors—(ZEB1; also known as deltaEF1) and SIP1 (also known as ZEB2) [34]. miR-200a is responsible for significant inhibition of cell proliferation and colony formation rate in HCCLM3 and HepG2 cell lines, while knocking out miR-200a restores the rate of proliferation and colony formation of cancer cells [35]. miRNA expression levels of miR-200 family tend to be decreased in individuals with liver cancer (plasma and tissue), compared with healthy individuals, and have a prognostic value for patients with HCC: microRNA-200a and miR-200c were independent prognostic factors for hepatocellular carcinoma and induced cell cycle arrest by targeting CDK6 or MAD2L1, respectively [36]. Opposite to miR-200 family, expression of miR-21 is induced in response to TGF-β signaling and is associated with tumor invasion and chemoresistance *in vitro*. Besides this, Wang Z et al. mention, indicating this is unpublished data, that Notch-1 could be one of miR-200b targets because overexpression of miR-200b significantly inhibited Notch-1 expression [37]. Moreover, miR-21 is able to directly interact with TGF-beta receptors: Mishra S. et al. revealed that miR-21 suppresses a tumor-suppressor gene TGFBR2 (transforming growth factor-beta receptor II) levels by binding to its 3 0-UTR, hence inhibiting the tumor-suppressive activity of TGFβ pathway [38]. Reported target genes for miR-21 in HCC are the following: FASLG, PTEN, HBP1, IL-12, RECK, and TIMP-3; some of these genes were shown simultaneously to be miR-21 targets in other liver diseases, such as ALD (FASLG), NAFLD (HBP1), and liver fibrosis (TIMP3) [39]. There are plenty of data showing an increase in miR-21 expression level in the background of liver cancer development or the chronic liver diseases, which are the risk factors for liver cancer development.

Members of the miR-17-92 and the miR-106b-25 clusters have been implicated in the progression of liver fibrosis through the influence on the expression of TGF-β receptor II (TGF-βRII), having opposite effects on this expression. miR-19b has been shown to play an inhibitory role in hepatic stem cell-mediated fibrogenesis and to be decreased in fibrotic rats and human livers. Overexpression of miR-19b inhibited the expression of TGF-βRII, which in turn inhibited SMAD3 expression and, as a result, reduced type-1 collagen production. Unlike miR-19b, miR-93 and miR-106b were observed to be consistently upregulated during the development of cirrhosis, and miR-106b along with miR-181was shown to have a diagnostic value for liver cirrhosis irrespective of the etiology [40].

miR-211, which is known to be involved in TGF-β interaction in prostate cancer cells, was shown to be involved in WNT-β signaling regulation via SATB2. In prostate cancer cells, increased expression of miR-211 inhibited expression of TGF-β1, TGF-β2, smad2, smad3, phosphorylated smad2, and smad3, and stem cell markers and *in vitro* resulted in reductions in the proliferation, invasion, colony-forming ability, sphere-forming ability, and stemness of prostate cancer stem cells, *in vivo* in decreased tumor growth, and cell apoptosis [41]. In HCC cells, miR-211 is supposed to suppress cancer cell proliferation *via* WNT-β and SATB2 downregulation. 3′-UTR of SATB2 was shown to be the direct target of miR-211, it contains a conserved target site for miR-211, and *in vitro* miR-211 mimics repressed the luciferase activity of the luciferase gene with inserted 3′-UTR of SATB2 in the pGL3-control vector. miR-211 expression in HCC tissues and cells is inversely correlated with SATB2, when in HCC tissues miR-211 expression was decreased, SATB2 expression was upregulated.

MiR-125b is known to interact with the Hh pathway, which is a well-known factor regulating liver reconstitution. miR-125b, produced by CP-MSCs (chorionic platelet-derived mesenchymal stem cells), attenuates Hh activation partly due to Smo expression inhibition and the consequence of this regulation is the promotion of the regression of fibrosis, contributing to liver regeneration [42]. It was demonstrated that another target of miR-125b in HCC cells is LIN28B, and simultaneously miR-125b may increase p21Cip1/Waf1 expression and arrest cell cycle at G_1 to S transition, which may contribute to suppression of HCC cell migration, invasion, and growth *in vitro* and *in vivo* [43]. With regard to this data, Liu W. et al. demonstrated that the expression level of serum exosomal miR-125b in patients with HCC (158 samples, qRT-PCR, normalization normalized to caenorhabditis elegans miRNA (Cel-miR-39)) was decreased in comparison with the expression level of serum exosomal miR-125b in patients with chronic hepatitis B (n=30) and liver cirrhosis (n=30). Moreover, the exosomal serum miR-125b level was shown to have a prognostic value for HCC patients: It predicted the recurrence and survival of HCC patients with an area under the ROC curve of 0.739 (83.0% sensitivity and 67.9% specificity) and 0.702 (82.5% sensitivity and 53.4% specificity) [44]. Moreover, inhibition of miR-125b suppressed the expression of profibrogenic genes in culture-activated primary HSCs and reduced the basal and transforming growth factor β (TGF-β)-induced alpha-smooth muscle actin (α-SMA) expression and cell contraction of the immortalized HSC cell line [45].

miRNA-199a-3p, being one of the putative therapeutic tools in liver cancer, may perform its anticancer effect through involvement in NOTCH signaling. miRNA-199a-3p is downregulated in liver cancer tissues and most liver cancer cell lines; in liver cancer cell lines (MHCC97H, Hep3B, SMMC-7721, Huh7, and HepG2), its expression was significantly lower than in normal liver cell lines; simultaneously, mRNA YAP1 expression was significantly higher than in normal liver cell lines. It was shown that miRNA-199a-3p targets YAP1, downregulates Jagged1, and suppresses the Notch signaling, which results in HCC cell proliferation inhibition and apoptosis promotion [46]. In a mouse model with induced HCC treatment with miRNA-199a-3p showed regression of hepatocellular carcinoma with the restoration of normal architecture on histopathological examination of liver specimens [47].

In liver cancer, HGF, ERBB3, and NF-κB form a positive feedback loop: higher expression of ERBB3 makes liver cancer cells more sensitive to HGF stimulation; moreover, HGF enhances ERBB3 expression by NF-κB transcriptional activity. miR-17-5p and miR-20a-5p in liver cancer cell lines and mice xenograft models were shown to suppress liver cancer cell proliferation after hepatectomy *via* blocking

HGF, ERBB3, and NF-κB positive feedback loop. HCC patients with lower levels of miR-17-5p and miR-20a-5p or higher levels of ERBB3 had significantly shorter OS and PFS survivals after surgical resection [48]. Simultaneous deregulation of VEFG and miRNA expression was shown in tissue samples of patients with liver cirrhosis, while VEGF did not show a significant difference in expression level in HCC samples compared to control (non-cancer and non-cirrhotic) samples. Expression level of VEGF was 12.97-fold higher in cirrhotic patients compared to liver cancer samples; concurrently, miR-206 and miR-637 (RT-qPCR, U6, RNU44, and RNU48 were used as reference genes) were down-expressed in LC samples. miR-637 was downregulated in HCC samples too [49]. Before it was shown that in HCC cells, miR-637 is responsible for suppressing autocrine leukemia inhibitory factor (LIF) expression and exogenous LIF-triggered activation of the transcription factor Stat3, which regulates several growth factors, including the VEGFA gene [50]. miR-146a indirectly influences VEGF expression in HCC cells through upregulating APC, which inhibits β-catenin accumulation in nucleus, and downregulating NF-κB p65 by targeting HAb18G [51]. An increase in expression of mRNA Jak2 and Stat3 along with reduced expression of miRNA-409 and reduction of Jak2 and Stat3 protein in response to miRNA-409 overexpression in liver cancer cells may allow to assume miRNA-409 in liver cancer playing an antitumor function through interaction with Jak2 and Stat3. Increased expression of miRNA-409 in liver cancer cells led to a decrease in cell viability and increased apoptosis. This miRNA expression level was significantly decreased in liver cancer tissues compared with paracancerous and normal liver tissues and was negatively correlated with tumor stage, tumor size, and overall survival time of patients with liver cancer [52]. Another miRNA, which is putatively involved in interaction with Jak2 and Stat3 in liver cancer, is miRNA-543, whose expression level was also shown to be decreased in liver cancer tissues. Like miRNA-409, it has a protective role in liver cancer and OS in patients with liver cancer and increased miRNA-543 is longer than in patients with decreased miRNA-543. Inhibition of miRNA-543 expression resulted in liver cancer cells with exactly the same consequences like inhibition of miRNA-409: increased cancer cell proliferation and decreased apoptosis. It also activated the protein expression of phosphorylated JAK2, phosphorylated STAT3, c-Myc, and B-cell lymphoma 2 (Bcl-2) in liver cancer cells [53]. miRNA-3662, which downregulated in HCC tissues and cell lines, may be involved in reprogramming cancer cells' glucose metabolism and forming of Warburg effect while having hypoxia-inducible factor-1α (HIF-1α) as one of the direct targets. Gain-of-function and loss-of-function assays showed that miR-3662 dampened glycolysis by reducing lactate production, glucose consumption, cellular glucose-6-phosphate level, ATP generation, and extracellular acidification rate, and increasing oxygen consumption rate in HCC cells [54]. Another putative target of miRNA-3662 in HCC cells, which allows its regulation of glucose metabolism, is hexokinase 2 (HK2). miR-3662 expression was decreased in liver cancer tissues and cells, while overexpression of miR-3662 or knockdown of HK2 inhibited cell proliferation, invasion, and glucose metabolism in cancer liver cells, which could be reversed by upregulating HK2 [55].

Taking into account the ambiguous relation between miRNA and mRNA expression levels and other factors, including circRNAs and proteins, associated with miRNA biogenesis and those involved in miRNA and mRNA interactions, prediction of changes in miRNA expression levels in any cancer, including liver cancer, becomes not that obvious task.

5. miRNAs and cancer cell metabolism

Along with changes on the genetic level, metabolic changes accompany cancer development in order to provide cells functioning in changing conditions, mainly hypoxia and glucose insufficiency due to intensive cell proliferation and clonal expansion and lagging in blood vessel formation. One of the main such metabolic reorganizations is Warburg effect, firstly reported in rat liver carcinoma in the 1920s and defined as an increase in the rate of glucose uptake and preferential production of lactate even in the presence of oxygen [56]. Main miRNAs, which are involved in Warburg effect realization in HCC cells, are miR-1, miR-122, and miR-338-3p [57]. The expression of the miR-1 targets G6PD and is mediated by NRF2, which, besides activating the transcription of genes encoding glycolytic enzymes, inhibits the conversion of pyruvate to acetyl-CoA by directly activating pyruvate dehydrogenase kinase 1 (PDK1) and leads to inhibition of tricarboxylic acid (TCA) cycle, promoting Warburg effect [58]. At the background of these interactions, it may appear to be regular that a higher expression of miR-1 showed a significant positive prognostic meaning for patients with HCC: Individuals with higher miR-1 serum levels showed longer OS than those with lower miR-1 serum concentrations (195 sera of HCC patients and 54 patients with liver cirrhosis; HR 0.451, 95% CI 0.228–0.856, $P = 0.015$). At the same time, serum miR-1 and miR-122 concentrations did not differ significantly between patients with HCC and liver cirrhosis [58].

miR-122 is another element of the processes that are assumed to restrain Warburg effect promotion, as far as among its main targets are Agpat 1 and Dgat 1 mRNAs, involved in triglyceride synthesis. One of the most important direct targets of miR-122 in HCC cells is PKM2, which is the most abundant pyruvate kinase iso-enzyme in liver tumors and a co-activator of several transcription factors, such as HIF-1α, β-catenin/c-Myc, NF-κB, and STAT3. Once in the nucleus, PKM2 can promote the transcription of target genes, such as HIF-1α targeted expression of GLUTs, PKM2, LDH-A, and VEGF-A, leading to the promotion of growth, positive feedback regulated glycolysis, and angiogenesis in cancer cells [59], and all these allow miR-122 to promote a decrease in lactate production and increase in oxygen consumption, thus reversing oxygen-independent glycolytic metabolism. Along with this, Yang G. et al. showed that miR-122 is downregulated in tissue samples from patients with HCC and also participates in ADAM17 regulation, which makes upregulation of miR-122 to inhibit proliferation of HCC cells *in vitro* [60]. In general, miR-122 is putatively one of the first examples of a tissue-specific miRNA and is highly expressed in the liver, where it constitutes 70% of the total miRNA pool [61]. Moreover, miR-122 has a prognostic role in HCC patients, and its downregulation is associated with poor prognosis: The overall survival time of the patients with low and high miR-122 expression in HCC was 30.3±8.0 and 83.7±10.3 months, respectively ($P<0.001$, tissue samples from 64 HCC patients and 28 matched non-neoplastic surrounding liver tissues) [62].

miR-338-3p has the same impact on Warburg effect in cancer liver cells such as miR-1 and miR-122, inhibiting it through decreasing expression of liver and red blood cell pyruvate kinase isoform (PKLR). miR-338-3p may be inactivated in HCC due to upregulation of circMAT2B, sequestering miR-338-3p due to its sponging activity, and disabling the regulation of its target gene PKM2 leading to increased proliferation, invasion, spheroid formation, and organoid dimensions, especially in hypoxic conditions [59]. Expression of miR-338-3p in tissue samples from patients with HCC was also shown to be decreased [33].

miR-23 was shown to be involved in gluconeogenesis regulation in liver cancer developed in the mouse model. Reduction in serum glucose in tumor-bearing mice correlated with a reduction in the expressions of G6pc, Pepck, and Fbp1 encoding the key gluconeogenic enzymes glucose-6-phosphatase, phosphoenolpyruvate carboxykinase, fructose-1,6-phosphatase, respectively, and the transcription factor Pgc-1α along with upregulation of miR-23a expression. mRNA levels of these genes were reduced to ≈80% in the majority of primary human HCC tissue samples compared with matching peritumoral liver samples and miR-23a was also upregulated in human liver cancer samples. Moreover, PGC-1α and G6PC expression negatively correlated with miR-23a expression in human HCCs [63]. miR-23a has a significant diagnostic value as far as it may distinguish cirrhotic liver samples from cancer liver samples, being higher in the HCC group than cirrhotic. miR-23a was significantly higher in HCC patients with focal lesion size equal or more than 5 cm, patients with multiple focal lesions, and Okuda stage III. At cutoff value ≥ 210, miR-23a showed accuracy of 79.3% to diagnose HCC patients with sensitivity of 89.47% and specificity of about 64.91% ((57 patients with HCC, 57 patients with liver cirrhosis (LC), and 57 healthy subjects as control group) and serum alpha-fetoprotein at cut off level ≥ 200 ng/mL had 73.68% sensitivity and 52.63% specificity for diagnosis of HCC [64].

6. Differential expression of miRNAs in chronic liver disease

Pathological states in some cases underlying liver cancer development are also accompanied by changes in miRNA expression levels such as hepatitis B virus infection, hepatitis C virus infection, nonalcoholic fatty liver disease (NAFLD), and alcoholic liver disease. One of miRNAs, which is associated with hepatitis virus, is miR-23 [31]. Other miRNAs also may differentiate HCC samples at the background of viral hepatitis from others, such as miR-17-92. Together with miR-21, its expression level was increased in hepatitis B virus-positive human and woodchuck HCC samples. Possibly, hepatitis B virus X and miR-17-92 share common target gene, which is c-myc, which is activated by virus and is known to be the instrument of carcinogenesis promotion of miR-17-92 [65]. Unlike HCV infection, HBV is known to induce HCC development gapping cirrhosis stage, thus making molecular predictors of cancer in this case especially required. Besides miR-122 and miR-17-92, other miRNAs, involved in HBV pathogenesis following HCC development, are miR-184, miR-185, miR-196a, miR-199a-3p, miR-210, miR-217, and miR-34a, which are involved in HBV transcription process. The expression of the last is inhibited by HBV X protein (HBx) *via* p53 stimulation in hepatocytes, upregulating a macrophage-derived chemokine (CCL22), participating in regulatory T cells stimulation and effector T cells suppression, which results in increasing HBV genome transcription [66, 67]. Another miRNA, whose expression changes in HBV infection due to HBx, is miR-155. Upregulation of miR-155 leads to a reduction in the suppressor of cytokine signaling-1 (SOCS1) expression, increasing JAK/STAT signaling and suppressing HBV infection mediated by the induction of interferon (IFN) signaling [68]. Some of these miRNAs, which are involved in HBV transcription process, are also involved in the regulation of signaling pathways, disrupted in the cancer development. Among putative targets of miRNA-199a-3p are mTOR, c-Met, HIF-1α, CD44, ROCK1, and Axl, so this miRNA, being downregulated in liver cancer samples, may inhibit cell proliferation, migration, and invasion [69]. miRNA-184 may function as an anti-apoptotic factor in liver cancer, and INPPL1 was identified as one of its targets. Through inhibition of the activities of caspases 3/7 and INPPL1 loss, it promotes cancer cell proliferation [70]. Similar function in HCC development through another target may play miRNA-196a. One of its direct targets is FOXO1, whose inhibition caused by miRNA-196a overexpression resulted in liver cancer cell migration and invasion *in vivo* [71]. miRNA-210 is known to be overexpressed in liver cancer samples and in HBV-associated liver cirrhosis; moreover, its expression was significantly higher in HepG2.2.15 cells than that in HepG2 cells. EGR3 was shown to be the target of miRNA-210, contrary to miRNA-210 the expression of EGR3 was downregulated in HBV-associated liver cirrhosis and liver cancer. In general, its role, like the role of miRNA-196a and miRNA-184, may be in proliferation promotion, and it is hard to assume whether the described mechanism with involvement in EGR3 regulation is specific for HBV-associated liver cancer, as far as EGR3 is known to be decreased in other cancers, like in head and neck cancers and gastric cancer [72]. miRNA-210 was also shown to be involved in bile acid-induced cholestatic liver injury through its direct target MLL4 (the histone methyltransferase mixed-lineage leukemia-4). miRNA-210 was the most highly elevated miR in mice with elevated hepatic BA levels and its expression was increased in patients with primary biliary cholangitis/cirrhosis (PBC) [73]. Opposite to the mentioned miRNAs, miRNA-217 inhibits liver cancer cell proliferation *via* targeting NAT2; moreover, its overexpression contributed to steatosis in hepatocytes as well as inflammation in mice, acting as a critical regulator in ethanol-induced hepatic inflammation [74]. miRNA-185 was shown to be involved in cholesterol metabolism in mouse model, and animals with knockout of this miRNA developed worsened hepatic steatosis upon high-fat high-cholesterol Western diet feeding with accumulation of triglyceride and cholesterol in the liver and developed hypercholesterolemia upon Western diet feeding. Treatment with miRNA-185 showed an improved accumulation of lipids in high-fat diet mouse model and insulin sensitivity *via* upregulation of the insulin-receptor substrate-2 [75, 76].

In case of HCV infection, there are miRNAs, which not just regulate expression of the genes, involved in virus replication, but are able to directly target the viral genome. Among these miRNAs are miR-196, miR-448, and miR-122, which stabilize the 5′ and 3′ UTRs of the HCV genome, so inhibition of this miRNA dramatically reduces the replication of HCV RNA [77, 78]. miRNAs, involved in viral replication *via* reducing tumor suppressor deleted in liver cancer 1 (DLC-1) and cell entry *via* the PI3K/AKT signaling pathway, are miR-141 and miR-491, respectively [76].

When it concerns alcoholic liver disease, miRNA expression profile changes especially due to increase in expression of inflammation-related miRNAs, such as miR-132, miR-155, miR-146, and miR-21, which influence alcohol/lipopolysaccharide (LPS)/TLR4 pathways, transmitting proinflammatory stimuli *via* a mitogen-activated protein kinases (MAPKs) or TIR domain-containing adaptor-inducing IFN-β (TRIF) [79, 80]. The imbalance between expression of let-7 and LIN28/28B has the crucial consequences, as far as regular alcohol overdose consumption diminishes let-7 expression, and loss of let-7 induces transformation of hepatic stellate cells (HSC) to mesenchymal phenotype, enhancing liver injury *via* inhibiting LIN28B, and thus promoting oncogenesis [81]. One of mechanisms underlying fibrosis formation in response to alcohol consumption is miR-34a, and its upregulation causes deregulation of its direct targets such as caspase-2, SIRT1, and matrix metallopeptidase (MMP) 1 and MMP2 [82].

Another risk factor for HCC development is NAFLD. It was revealed that miR-34a and miR-122 identified in blood serum are potential markers for discriminating NAFLD patients from healthy controls with an area under the curve (AUC) values of 0.781 and 0.858, respectively, along with miR-21, miR-125b, and miR-375 did not show significant difference in level expression between NAFLD patients and healthy controls. Serum levels of miR-34a and miR-122 were found to be significantly higher among NAFLD patients and were positively correlated with VLDL-C and triglyceride levels [83]. The other study showed the same tendency for miRNA-34a and miRNA-122, and also found a significant difference in level expression of following miRNA: miR-21and miR-451. Moreover, the serum level of miR-122 was correlated with the severity of liver steatosis; however, in the previous study, the expression levels of miR-34a and miR-122 did not correlate with the histological features of NAFLD [83]. There is at least one common signaling pathway, involving both miRNA-34a and miRNA-122, which is AMPK [21, 82]. It should be admitted that along with being possibly involved in the regulation of the same targets, miRNA-122 and miRNA-34 definitely should have similar effects as far as miRNA-122 expression is decreased in cancers including liver cancer, and miRNA-34 expression is decreased in liver cancer while being elevated in chronic hepatitis C patients. Targets and mechanisms of miRNA-34 involvement in the liver cancer development are known in less details than miRNA-122. It is supposed, that through involvement in the Sirt1/p53 pathway regulation, miRNA-34 promotes liver fibrosis in patients with HCV [84]. It is possible to speculate that with loss of the benign liver cells phenotype, malignant liver cells lose possibility of normal miRNA-34 expression as far as miRNA-34 expression is significantly decreased in liver cancer cells. One of the possible mechanisms of miRNA-34 involvement in the liver cancer development is glucose metabolism, in which LDHA, which is the target gene of miRNA-34, participates in glucose metabolism reprograming with its switch to the increased glycolysis [85]. In its turn, miRNA-122 is also indirectly involved in glucose metabolism, having Igf1R as one of its targets [63]. The other putative intersection of these two miRNAs is p53 pathway, as far as both participate in its regulation. miRNA-34 in the context of HCV fibrosis via Sirt1 regulation and miRNA-122 through cyclin G1, which results in increased p53 protein stability activity and reduction in invasion capabilities of HCC cells with elevated miRNA-122 expression [86]. Another miRNA-132, which possibly shares with miRNA-34 SIRT1 as a common target, is miRNA-132. This miRNA is elevated in the response to alcohol consumption, while *in vivo* and *in vitro* studies suggest miR-132 targets SIRT1, being increased in HCC cells and associated with unfavorable survival in HCC patients [87].

With the cancer development, differences in miRNA expression profiles smooth out as far as cancer cell phenotype and functions despite its different background development including such common features as promoted proliferation, disrupted apoptosis, and increased migratory and invasion capabilities. miRNA expression during the process of malignization changes in conformity with these demands, so far miRNA-34, being elevated in HCV liver cirrhosis, is decreased in the liver cancer cells. Obviously, all changes in miRNA expression during cancer development tend to upregulation of oncogenic miRNAs and downregulation of tumor suppressor miRNAs, and with evolution of the stage of the tumor differences in miRNA expression associated with different background liver disease level out. However, different miRNAs may be involved in the same signaling pathways or share common target genes, which is allowed by the sequence and molecular nature of miRNA—mRNA interaction—and indirect influence of miRNA on the expression levels of the genes, which are not its direct targets.

7. Differential expression of miRNAs in HCC

Concerning signaling pathways disrupted in HCC, almost all these pathways the regulation is double-sided: miRNA may regulate the expression of the genes and genes may regulate the expression of miRNAs. For example, TGF-β signaling may modulate miRNA expression level *via* canonical pathway, which is Smad-dependent requiring co-Smad Smad4, and non-canonical pathway, such as Smad4-independent. The Smad binding element found in the promoters of TGF-β/BMP-regulated genes contains a conserved sequence similar to the pre-miRNAs of TGF-β/BMP-regulated miRNAs, which is CAGAC [88]. miRNAs, containing this RNA-Smad binding element (R-SBE), are following: miR-105, miR-199a, miR-215, miR-421, and miR-529 [34]. The miRNAs upregulated by TGF-β signaling include miR-21, the miR-181 family, miR-10b, the miR-17/92 cluster, miR-155, miR-192, the miR-23/24/27 cluster, miR-216/217, miR-494, and miR-182. The miRNAs downregulated by TGF-β signaling include the miR-200 family, miR-203, let-7, miR-34a, and miR-584 [34]. Many miRNAs targeting different substrates of TGF-β pathway are frequently oncogenic, such as miR-200, having impact on the expression of TGF-β ligands and TGF-β receptors type I and II, miR-21, miR0211, miR-17/92, and miR-106b/206, mainly participating in regulation of expression TGF-β receptors type I and II and miR-182, involved in the regulation of R-Smad, co-Smad (I-Smad), and Smad7, and it modulates a negative feedback loop of TGF-β signaling as Smad7 is also induced by TGF-β. Besides TGF-β receptors type I and II, miR-17/92 and miR-106b/205 participate in the regulation of downstream targets of TGF-β pathway [34].

miR-141 and miR-200a expression levels were shown to be decreased and serum samples from patients with liver cancer (blood samples were taken from 30 patients with liver cancer and from 30 normal subjects, RNU6 or GAPDH as internal controls). The sensitivity and specificity of the investigated miRNAs for diagnosing tumor invasion in liver cancer and comparing metastasis of patients with liver cancer were higher in combination of miR-141 and miR-200a rather than alone, although the difference between AUC values in both cases—combination and one miR regimen—had no significant changes. The possible mechanism of cancer processes modulation was explained with E-cadherin and vimentin inhibition due to STAT4 inhibition, which was firstly reported as a target gene for these miRNAs [89, 90]. The study of Dhayat et al. also showed a significant negative correlation of miR-200a and miR-200b to the expression of the mesenchymal markers Vimentin and ZEB-1 and a significant positive correlation to the epithelial marker E-cadherin. Moreover, in this study, miR-200 family was significantly downregulated in HCC samples compared to liver cirrhosis and was shown to be able to distinguish between cirrhotic and HCC tissue [90].

miR-211-5p was significantly downregulated in patients with HCC (30 pairs of HCC tissues and matched adjacent tumor-free tissues, qRT-PCR, RNU6 (miRNA) as an endogenous control), although miR-211-5p expression in liver cancer samples was not significantly different from adjacent normal samples based on TCGA cohorts, it was considerably downregulated in 30 pairs of HCC tissues compared with matched adjacent tumor-free tissues from patients in clinics or real-world cohorts. It was also shown that miR-211-5p may have a prognostic role for HCC patients: Patients with a decreased expression of miR-211-5p had poor overall survival [91]. In another study, miR-211-5p was found to be decreased in 33 out of 40 HCC tissue samples compared with the corresponding non-tumor tissues; moreover, tissues from lymph node metastases also expressed lower levels of miR-211 compared with primary HCC tissues and the adjacent normal tissue (qRT-PCR, the endogenous U6 snRNA or GAPDH as the internal control) [68]. Among miR-211-5p targets are STAB2, SPARC, ZEB2, and ACSL4, negatively regulating these genes, miR-211-5p participates in the suppression of cell proliferation, migration, and invasion in HCC tissues [92].

In contrast, miR-17/92 expression levels were shown to be highly expressed in HCC tissues compared to the non-tumor liver tissues (94 cases of HCC, 5 cases of cancer adjacent to normal hepatic tissue, and 5 cases of normal liver tissue; U6 small nuclear 2 (U6b) as an internal control, RT-PCR). In this study, it was shown that expression of miR-17-92 was negatively correlated with several target genes, including CREBL2, PRRG1, and NTN4, when analyzing the miRNA and mRNA sequencing data from the 312 hepatocellular cancer patients available from the TCGA database [68].

Expression level of miR-182-5p was also elevated in HCC tissues and its high expression level correlated with poor prognosis such as early recurrence in patients who underwent curative surgery (tissue samples from 119 patients; RT-PCR, U6 snRNA was probed as a loading control; the disease-free survival was calculated from the date of resection to the date of tumor recurrence). Promotion of HCC proliferation by miR-182-5p is partly possible due to the ability of the last to directly target 3′-UTR of FOXO3a and thus inhibits FOXO3a expression, activating AKT/FOXO3a pathway. MiR-182-5p interacts with 3`-UTR of FOXO3a by binding to the 72-79 site, but not the 914–921 site in the 3′-UTR of FOXO3a [93].

However, in almost all these pathways the regulation is double-sided: miRNA may regulate the expression of the genes, and genes may regulate the expression of miRNAs. TGF-β signaling may modulate miRNA expression level *via* the canonical pathway, which is Smad-dependent requiring co-Smad Smad4, and non-canonical pathway, such as Smad4-independent. The Smad binding element found in the promoters of TGF-β/BMP-regulated genes contains a conserved sequence similar to the pre-miRNAs of TGF-β/BMP-regulated miRNAs, which is CAGAC [34]. miRNAs, containing this RNA-Smad binding element (R-SBE), are following: miR-105, miR-199a, miR-215, miR-421, and miR-529 [34]. The miRNAs upregulated by TGF-β signaling include miR-21, the miR-181 family, miR-10b, the miR-17/92 cluster, miR-155, miR-192, the miR-23/24/27 cluster, miR-216/217, miR-494, and miR-182. The miRNAs downregulated by TGF-β signaling include the miR-200 family, miR-203, let-7, miR-34a, and miR-584 [34]. Many miRNAs targeting different substrates of TGF-β pathway are frequently oncogenic, such as miR-200, having an impact on the expression of TGF-β ligands and TGF-β receptors type I and II, miR-21, miR0211, miR-17/92, and miR-106b/206, mainly participating in regulation of expression TGF-β receptors type I and II and miR-182, involved in regulation of R-Smad and co-Smad (I-Smad) and Smad7, and it modulates a negative feedback loop of TGF-β signaling as Smad7 is also induced by TGF-β. Besides TGF-β receptors type I and II, miR-17/92 and miR-106b/205 participate in regulation of downstream targets of TGF-β pathway [34].

It may seem interesting that almost none of these miRNAs were included in the list of miRNAs, implying HCC signature based on TCGA database, which consists of 540 miRNA expression profiles from 348 HCC patients, of whom 248 had early-stage and 90 had advanced-stage HCC. SVM-HCC, based on an SVM29 incorporating the feature selection algorithm IBCGAa proposed method, used a feature selection algorithm (IBCGA) to select a significant miRNA signature associated with early and advanced stages of HCC. This signature contains 23 miRNAs: in order of decreasing MED (Main

Effect Difference) scores, miR-550a, miR-549, miR-518b, miR-512, miR-1179, miR-574, miR-424, miR-4286, let-7i, miR-320a, miR-17, miR-299, miR-3651, miR-2277, miR-621, miR-181c, miR-539, miR-106b, miR-1269, miR-139, miR-152, miR-2355, and miR-150. Moreover, the significance of 10 top-ranked miRNAs in distinguishing HCC tissue samples from normal tissue samples and their prognostic values were proved on different datasets [94]. For some of these miRNAs with the highest MED scores, there are known targets in the context of liver cancer development. Among direct targets of miRNA-320a, there are β-catenin, c-myc, cyclin D1, and dickkopf-1; functional studies have shown a significantly decreased capability of cell proliferation and G0/G1 growth arrest *in vitro* when miRNA-320 is overexpressed [95]. miRNA-424 demonstrated a strong prognostic value in liver cancer: Its expression level in HCC tissues was associated with a relapse after liver transplantation. The study involved samples from 121 patients, the median follow-up duration was 25.12 months, U6 snRNA was used as the endogenous control [96]. In liver cancer cell lines, it was shown that miRNA-574-3p has an ADAM28 as a direct target and binds 3′-untranslated region of the ADAM28 mRNA leading to reduced cell proliferation and migration and promoted cell apoptosis [97]. Like miRNA-200 and miRNA-211-5p, which are mentioned above in the context of HCC development and which are not listed in this miRNA list, miRNA-1179 directly interacts with zinc-finger E-box-binding homeobox 2 (ZEB2) and has antitumor function, leading to attenuated proliferation and migration of HCC cells. Its expression was decreased in HCC tissues compared with corresponding noncancerous tissues (40 paired HCC samples with matched normal tissues, U6 were used as internal reference) [98]. miRNA-550a plays a controversial role in HCC development, promoting HCC cell migration and invasion, and cytoplasmic polyadenylation element-binding protein 4 (CPEB4) is one of its potential targets, which is commonly decreased in liver cancer. The function of CPEB4, which is from the gene family CPEB involved in regulation of translation by controlling the polyadenylation of target genes, is yet to be elucidated. There are contradictional data of its function in cancer development: In pancreatic ductal cancer and neuroblastoma, its expression is upregulated, driving the growth and invasion of cancer cells. In HCC, it was shown that CPEB4 siRNA could promote the migration and invasion of HCC cells. This contradiction may be explained by different downstream targets regulated by CPEB4 in different cells because CPEB4 along with involvement in polyadenylation can control the translation by binding to the CPE sequence in 3′ UTR of the corresponding genes [99]. miRNA-512 may play one of the crucial roles in HCC progression, being significantly upregulated in human HCC samples and HCC cell lines. Along with miRNA-519, it targets tumor suppressors MAP3K2 and MAP2K4, and the integration of these two miRNAs into the AJCC staging system significantly improved the accuracy of the prediction of HCC recurrence [100]. Some of these miRNAs, such as miRNA-518b, miRNA-549, miRNA-2277, and miRNA-2355, are rarely mentioned in the context of liver cancer development, and their role in this process is yet to be elucidated.

This emphasizes the importance of working with customized algorithms and validated big datasets, when many of the aspects of the process you are studying—like miRNA involvement in carcinogenesis—stay unclear, making identification of the most promising diagnostic and/or prognostic and/or therapeutic molecules *via* analyzing only mRNA-miRNA interactions or miRNAs in signaling or metabolic pathways not very effective.

In **Table 1**, there are listed miRNAs, whose expression levels are changed in the HCC development in order of mention in the text.

No.	miRNA	Decreased or increased compared with normal tissue	Possible targets	Effects of overexpression	References
1	miRNA-200a	Decreased	ZEB1, ZEB2, TGF-β	Inhibition of cell proliferation and colony formation rate	[34, 35]
2	miRNA-21	Increased	TGFBR2 FASLG, PTEN, HBP1, IL-12, RECK, and TIMP-3	Promotion of tumor invasion and metastasis	[37, 39]
3	miR-211	Decreased	WNT-β signaling regulation *via* SATB2	Inhibition of cancer cells proliferation	[41]
4	miR-125b	Decreased	Hh	Arrest cell cycle at G_1 to S transition	[43, 44]
5	miRNA-199a-3p	Decreased	NOTCH, YAP1	Inhibition of HCC cell proliferation and induction of HCC cell apoptosis	[46]
6	miRNA-17-5p	Decreased	ERBB3	Inhibition of cancer cell proliferation	[48]
7	miRNA-637	Decreased	Autocrine leukemia inhibitory factor (LIF), Stat 3	Inhibition of cancer proliferation	[50]
8	miRNA-409	Decreased	Jak2, STAT3	Decreased cancer cell viability and increased apoptosis	[52]
9	miRNA-543	Decreased	Jak2, Stat3	Decreased cancer cell viability and increased apoptosis	[53]
10	miRNA-3662	Decreased	HIF-1α, HK2	Glucose metabolism transformation to Warburg effect, decreased glycolysis	[54, 55]
11	miRNA-122	Decreased	Agpat 1, Dgat1, PKM2, ADAM17	Inhibition of cancer cells proliferation	[59, 60]
12	miRNA-338-3p	Decreased	PKLR	Inhibition of Warburg effect	[30, 33]
13	miRNA-23	Increased	G6pc, Pepck, and Fbp1	Increased gluconeogenesis	[63]
14	miRNA-184	Increased	INPPL1	Promoting cancer cells proliferation	[70]
15	miRNA-196a	Increased	FOXO1	Promotion of liver cancer cell migration and invasion	[71]
16	miRNA-210	Increased	EGR3, MLL4	Promotion of liver cancer cell proliferation	[72, 73]
17	miRNA-217	Decreased	NAT2	Inhibition of cancer cell proliferation	[74]

No.	miRNA	Decreased or increased compared with normal tissue	Possible targets	Effects of overexpression	References
18	miRNA-34	Decreased	AMPK, Sirt1/p53, LDHA	Inhibition of gluconeogenesis	[85]
19	miRNA-122	Decreased	AMPK, Cyclin G1	Promotion of cancer cells proliferation	[86]
20	miRNA-132	Increased	SIRT1	Promotion of cancer cell proliferation	[87]
21	miRNA-141	Decreased	STAT4	Promotion of cancer cell proliferation	[89]
22	miRNA-17/92	Increased	CREBL2, PRRG1, NTN4	Promotion of cancer cell proliferation and invasion	[68]
23	miRNA-182-5p	Increased	FOXO3a	Promotion of cancer cell proliferation and invasion	[93]
24	miRNA-320a	Decreased	β-catenin, c-myc, cyclin D1 and dickkopf-1	Decreased capability of cell proliferation and G0/G1 growth arrest	[95]
25	miRNA-574-3p	Decreased	ADAM28	Reduced cancer cell proliferation and migration	[97]
26	miRNA-1179	Decreased	ZEB2	Reduced cancer cell proliferation and migration	[98]
27	miRNA-550a	Increased	CPEB4	Promotion of cancer cell proliferation	[99]
28	miRNA-512	Increased	MAP3K2, MAP2K4	Increased cancer cell proliferation rate and migration capability	[100]

Table 1.
miRNAs in liver cancer development.

8. Conclusion

miRNAs play a pivotal role in liver cancer development; presumably in the early stages of HCC development, its multiple miRNA expression profiles may be distinguished depending on the etiological factor, such as HBV, HCV, NAFLD, or ALD. miRNAs are biomarkers with a huge potency as far as they are small, stable, and protected from RNases *via* protein binding or exosome membrane and their expression level change at the background of metabolism and signaling pathways modification during malignancy in the liver. Biogenesis of miRNA and its interaction with mRNA are not clear and involve different proteins and other noncoding miRNAs, which make it difficult to predict miRNAs expression level change in the specific cancer type and require special algorithm and big data sets. It should be noted that changes in expression levels of almost all miRNAs listed above are not specific to liver cancer and are identified in prostate cancer, gastric cancer, colon cancer, and other cancer types. In this context, a multiple miRNA panel is a promising option for diagnostic purposes.

Conflict of interest

The authors declare no conflict of interest.

Author details

Alisa Petkevich*, Aleksandr Abramov and Vadim Pospelov
Scientific and Practical Center of Specialized Health Care for Children named after V.F. Voino-Yasenetskiy, Moscow, Russia

*Address all correspondence to: pa.alisa26@gmail.com

References

[1] Leitão AL, Enguita FJ. A structural view of miRNA biogenesis and function. Noncoding RNA. 2022;**8**(1):10. DOI: 10.3390/ncrna8010010

[2] Chou CH, Shrestha S, Yang CD, Chang NW, Lin YL, Liao KW, et al. miRTarBase update 2018: A resource for experimentally validated microRNA-target interactions. Nucleic Acids Research. 2018;**46**(D1):D296-D302. DOI: 10.1093/nar/gkx1067

[3] Bray F, Ferlay J, Soerjomataram I, Siegel RL, Torre LA, Jemal A, et al. GLOBOCAN estimates of incidence and mortality worldwide for 36 cancers in 185 countries. CA: A Cancer Journal for Clinicians. 2018;**2018**(68):394-424. DOI: 10.3322/caac.21492

[4] O'Brien J, Hayder H, Zayed Y, Peng C. Overview of microRNA biogenesis, mechanisms of actions, and circulation. Front Endocrinol (Lausanne). 2018;**9**:402. DOI: 10.3389/fendo.2018.00402

[5] Ha M, Kim VN. Regulation of microRNA biogenesis. Nature Reviews. Molecular Cell Biology. 2014;**15**:509-524. DOI: 10.1038/nrm3838

[6] Adams L. Non-coding RNA: Pri-miRNA processing: Structure is key. Nature Reviews. Genetics. 2017;**18**(3):145. DOI: 10.1038/nrg.2017.6

[7] Michlewski G, Guil S, Semple CA, Cáceres JF. Posttranscriptional regulation of miRNAs harboring conserved terminal loops. Molecular Cell. 2008;**32**(3):383-393. DOI: 10.1016/j.molcel.2008.10.013

[8] Yi R, Qin Y, Macara IG, Cullen BR. Exportin-5 mediates the nuclear export of pre-microRNAs and short hairpin RNAs. Genes & Development. 2003;**17**:3011-3016. DOI: 10.1101/gad.1158803

[9] Olena AF, Patton JG. Genomic organization of microRNAs. Journal of Cellular Physiology. 2010;**222**(3):540-545. DOI: 10.1002/jcp.21993

[10] Stavast CJ, Erkeland SJ. The non-canonical aspects of MicroRNAs: Many roads to gene regulation. Cell. 2019;**8**(11):1465. DOI: 10.3390/cells8111465

[11] Arora S, Rana R, Chhabra A, Jaiswal A, Rani V. miRNA-transcription factor interactions: A combinatorial regulation of gene expression. Molecular Genetics and Genomics. 2013;**288**(3-4):77-87. DOI: 10.1007/s00438-013-0734-z

[12] Martinez NJ, Walhout AJ. The interplay between transcription factors and microRNAs in genome-scale regulatory networks. BioEssays. 2009;**31**(4):435-445. DOI: 10.1002/bies.200800212

[13] Mullany LE, Herrick JS, Wolff RK, Stevens JR, Samowitz W, Slattery ML. MicroRNA-transcription factor interactions and their combined effect on target gene expression in colon cancer cases. Genes, Chromosomes & Cancer. 2018;**57**(4):192-202. DOI: 10.1002/gcc.22520

[14] Zhou L, Miller C, Miraglia LJ, Romero A, Mure LS, Panda S, et al. A genome-wide microRNA screen identifies the microRNA-183/96/182 cluster as a modulator of circadian rhythms. Proceedings of the National Academy Science USA.

2021;**118**(1):e2020454118. DOI: 10.1073/pnas.2020454118

[15] Thomson DW, Dinger ME. Endogenous microRNA sponges: Evidence and controversy. Nature Reviews. Genetics. 2016;**17**(5):272-283. DOI: 10.1038/nrg.2016.20

[16] Plotnikova O, Baranova A, Skoblov M. Comprehensive analysis of human microRNA–mRNA interactome. Frontiers in Genetics. 2019;**10**:1-11. DOI: 10.3389/fgene.2019.00933

[17] Kersten S. Integrated physiology and systems biology of PPARα. Molecular Metabolism. 2014;**3**(4):354-371. DOI: 10.1016/j.molmet.2014.02.002

[18] Ding J, Li M, Wan X, Jin X, Chen S, Yu C, et al. Effect of miR-34a in regulating steatosis by targeting PPARα expression in nonalcoholic fatty liver disease. Scientific Reports. 2015;**5**:13729. DOI: 10.1038/srep13729

[19] Chai C, Rivkin M, Berkovits L, Simerzin A, Zorde-Khvalevsky E, Rosenberg N, et al. Metabolic circuit involving free fatty acids, microRNA 122, and triglyceride synthesis in liver and muscle tissues. Gastroenterology. 2017;**153**(5):1404-1415. DOI: 10.1053/j.gastro.2017.08.013

[20] Krützfeldt J, Rajewsky N, Braich R, Rajeev KG, Tuschl T, Manoharan M, et al. Silencing of microRNAs in vivo with 'antagomirs'. Nature. 2005;**438**(7068):685-689. DOI: 10.1038/nature04303

[21] Esau C, Davis S, Murray SF, Yu XX, Pandey SK, Pear M, et al. miR-122 regulation of lipid metabolism revealed by in vivo antisense targeting. Cell Metabolism. 2006;**3**(2):87-98. DOI: 10.1016/j.cmet.2006.01.005

[22] Chung HH. New insights for controversial issues of miR-122 in hepatic lipid metabolism. Gastroenterology. 2018;**154**(5):1552-1553. DOI: 10.1053/j.gastro.2017.12.039

[23] Morishita A, Oura K, Tadokoro T, Fujita K, Tani J, Masaki T. MicroRNAs in the pathogenesis of hepatocellular carcinoma: A review. Cancers (Basel). 2021;**13**(3):514. DOI: 10.3390/cancers13030514

[24] Ramírez CM, Goedeke L, Rotllan N, Yoon JH, Cirera-Salinas D, Mattison JA, et al. MicroRNA 33 regulates glucose metabolism. Molecular and Cellular Biology. 2013;**33**(15):2891-2902. DOI: 10.1128/MCB.00016-13

[25] Wu H, Zhang T, Pan F, Steer CJ, Li Z, Chen X, et al. MicroRNA-206 prevents hepatosteatosis and hyperglycemia by facilitating insulin signaling and impairing lipogenesis. Journal of Hepatology. 2017;**66**(4):816-824. DOI: 10.1016/j.jhep.2016.12.016

[26] Suksangrat T, Phannasil P, Jitrapakdee S. miRNA regulation of glucose and lipid metabolism in relation to diabetes and non-alcoholic fatty liver disease. Advances in Experimental Medicine and Biology. 2019;**1134**:129-148. DOI: 10.1007/978-3-030-12668-1_7

[27] Lotterman CD, Kent OA, Mendell JT. Functional integration of microRNAs into oncogenic and tumor suppressor pathways. Cell Cycle. 2008;**7**(16):2493-2499. DOI: 10.4161/cc.7.16.6452

[28] Pu J, Wang J, Li W, et al. Hsa_circ_0000092 promotes hepatocellular carcinoma progression through up-regulating HN1 expression by binding to microRNA-338-3p. Journal of Cellular and Molecular Medicine. 2020:1-13. DOI: 10.1111/jcmm.15010

[29] Liu Z, Yang D, Li Y, Jiao Y, Lv G. HN1 as a diagnostic and prognostic biomarker for liver cancer. Bioscience Reports. 2020;**40**(7):BSR20200316. DOI: 10.1042/BSR20200316

[30] Li Q, Pan X, Zhu D, Deng Z, Jiang R, Wang X. Circular RNA MAT2B promotes glycolysis and malignancy of hepatocellular carcinoma through the miR-338-3p/PKM2 axis under hypoxic stress. Hepatology. 2019;**70**(4):1298-1316. DOI: 10.1002/hep.30671

[31] Louis C, Leclerc D, Coulouarn C. Emerging roles of circular RNAs in liver cancer. JHEP Reports. 2021;**4**(2):100413. DOI: 10.1016/j.jhepr.2021.100413

[32] Liu J, Liu T, Wang X, He A. Circles reshaping the RNA world: From waste to treasure. Molecular Cancer. 2017;**16**(1):58. DOI: 10.1186/s12943-017-0630-y

[33] Suzuki HI. MicroRNA control of TGF-β signaling. International Journal of Molecular Sciences. 2018;**19**(7):1901. DOI: 10.3390/ijms19071901

[34] Gregory PA, Bracken CP, Smith E, et al. An autocrine TGF-beta/ZEB/miR-200 signaling network regulates establishment and maintenance of epithelial-mesenchymal transition. Molecular Biology of the Cell. 2011;**22**(10):1686-1698. DOI: 10.1091/mbc.E11-02-0103

[35] Feng J, Wang J, Chen M, et al. miR-200a suppresses cell growth and migration by targeting MACC1 and predicts prognosis in hepatocellular carcinoma. Oncology Reports. 2015;**33**:713-720. DOI: 10.3892/or.2014.3642

[36] Mao Y, Chen W, Wu H, Liu C, Zhang J, Chen S. Mechanisms and functions of MiR-200 family in hepatocellular carcinoma. Oncotargets and Therapy. 2021;**13**:13479-13490. DOI: 10.2147/OTT.S288791

[37] Wang Z, Li Y, Kong D, Ahmad A, Banerjee S, Sarkar FH. Cross-talk between miRNA and Notch signaling pathways in tumor development and progression. Cancer Letters. 2010;**292**(2):141-148. DOI: 10.1016/j.canlet.2009.11.012

[38] Mishra S, Deng JJ, Gowda PS, et al. Androgen receptor and microRNA-21 axis downregulates transforming growth factor beta receptor II (TGFBR2) expression in prostate cancer. Oncogene. 2014;**33**(31):4097-4106. DOI: 10.1038/onc.2013.374

[39] Zhang T, Yang Z, Kusumanchi P, Han S, Liangpunsakul S. Critical role of microRNA-21 in the pathogenesis of liver diseases. Front Med (Lausanne). 2020;**7**:7. DOI: 10.3389/fmed.2020.00007

[40] Tan W, Li Y, Lim SG, Tan TM. miR-106b-25/miR-17-92 clusters: Polycistrons with oncogenic roles in hepatocellular carcinoma. World Journal of Gastroenterology. 2014;**20**(20):5962-5972. DOI: 10.3748/wjg.v20.i20.5962

[41] Zhao Z, Wang K, Tan S. microRNA-211-mediated targeting of the INHBA-TGF-β axis suppresses prostate tumor formation and growth. Cancer Gene Therapy. 2021;**28**(5):514-528. DOI: 10.1038/s41417-020-00237-w

[42] Hyun J, Wang S, Kim J, et al. MicroRNA125b-mediated Hedgehog signaling influences liver regeneration by chorionic plate-derived mesenchymal stem cells. Scientific Reports. 2015;**5**:14135. DOI: 10.1038/srep14135

[43] Liang L, Wong CM, Ying Q, et al. MicroRNA-125b suppressesed human liver cancer cell proliferation and

metastasis by directly targeting oncogene LIN28B2. Hepatology. 2010;**52**(5): 1731-1740. DOI: 10.1002/hep.23904

[44] Liu W, Hu J, Zhou K, et al. Serum exosomal miR-125b is a novel prognostic marker for hepatocellular carcinoma. Oncotargets and Therapy. 2017;**10**:3843-3851. DOI: 10.2147/OTT.S140062

[45] You K, Li SY, Gong J, et al. MicroRNA-125b promotes hepatic stellate cell activation and liver fibrosis by activating RhoA signaling. Molecular Therapy--Nucleic Acids. 2018;**12**:57-66. DOI: 10.1016/j.omtn.2018.04.016

[46] Ren K, Li T, Zhang W, Ren J, Li Z, Wu G. miR-199a-3p inhibits cell proliferation and induces apoptosis by targeting YAP1, suppressing Jagged1-Notch signaling in human hepatocellular carcinoma. Journal of Biomedical Science. 2016;**23**(1):79. DOI: 10.1186/s12929-016-0295-7

[47] Atta S, Kramani NE, Mohamed SR, et al. MicroRNA-199: A potential therapeutic tool for hepatocellular carcinoma in an experimental model. Asian Pacific Journal of Cancer Prevention. 2021;**22**(9):2771-2779. DOI: 10.31557/APJCP.2021.22.9.2771

[48] Liu DL, Lu LL, Dong LL, et al. miR-17-5p and miR-20a-5p suppress postoperative metastasis of hepatocellular carcinoma via blocking HGF/ERBB3-NF-κB positive feedback loop. Theranostics. 2020;**10**(8):3668-3683. DOI: 10.7150/thno.41365

[49] de Oliveira ARCP, Castanhole-Nunes MMU, Biselli-Chicote PM, et al. Differential expression of angiogenesis-related miRNAs and VEGFA in cirrhosis and hepatocellular carcinoma. Archives of Medical Science. 2020;**16**(5):1150-1157. DOI: 10.5114/aoms.2020.97967

[50] Zhang JF, He ML, Fu WM, et al. Primate-specific microRNA-637 inhibits tumorigenesis in hepatocellular carcinoma by disrupting signal transducer and activator of transcription 3 signaling. Hepatology. 2011;**54**(6):2137-2148. DOI: 10.1002/hep.24595

[51] Zhang Z, Zhang Y, Sun XX, Ma X, Chen ZN. microRNA-146a inhibits cancer metastasis by downregulating VEGF through dual pathways in hepatocellular carcinoma. Molecular Cancer. 2015;**14**:5. DOI: 10.1186/1476-4598-14-5

[52] Zhang CS, Lin Y, Sun FB, Gao J, Han B, Li SJ. miR-409 down-regulates Jak-Stat pathway to inhibit progression of liver cancer. European Review for Medical and Pharmacological Sciences. 2019;**23**(1):146-154. DOI: 10.26355/eurrev_201901_16758

[53] Xiu D, Wang D, Wang J, Ji F, Zhang W. MicroRNA-543 suppresses liver cancer growth and induces apoptosis via the JAK2/STAT3 signaling pathway. Oncology Letters. 2019;**17**(2):2451-2456. DOI: 10.3892/ol.2018.9838

[54] Chen Z, Zuo X, Zhang Y, et al. MiR-3662 suppresses hepatocellular carcinoma growth through inhibition of HIF-1α-mediated Warburg effect. Cell Death & Disease. 2018;**9**(5):549. DOI: 10.1038/s41419-018-0616-8

[55] Ye J, Xiao X, Han Y, Fan D, Zhu Y, Yang L. MiR-3662 suppresses cell growth, invasion and glucose metabolism by targeting HK2 in hepatocellular carcinoma cells. Neoplasma. 2020;**67**(4):773-781. DOI: 10.4149/neo_2020_190730N689

[56] Farzaneh Z, Vosough M, Agarwal T, Farzaneh M. Critical signaling pathways governing hepatocellular carcinoma behavior; small molecule-based approaches. Cancer Cell International.

2021;**21**(1):208. DOI: 10.1186/s12935-021-01924-w

[57] Liberti MV, Locasale JW. The Warburg effect: How does it benefit cancer cells? Trends in Biochemical Sciences. 2016;**41**(3):211-218. DOI: 10.1016/j.tibs.2015.12.001

[58] Chang CW, Chen YS, Tsay YG, Han CL, Chen YJ, Yang CC, et al. ROS-independent ER stress-mediated NRF2 activation promotes warburg effect to maintain stemness-associated properties of cancer-initiating cells. Cell Death & Disease. 2018;**9**(2):194. DOI: 10.1038/s41419-017-0250-x

[59] Gramantieri L, Giovannini C, Piscaglia F, Fornari F. MicroRNAs as modulators of tumor metabolism, microenvironment, and immune response in hepatocellular carcinoma. Journal of Hepatocellular Carcinoma. 2021;**8**:369-385. DOI: 10.2147/JHC.S268292

[60] Köberle V, Kronenberger B, Pleli T, Trojan J, Imelmann E, Peveling-Oberhag J, et al. Serum microRNA-1 and microRNA-122 are prognostic markers in patients with hepatocellular carcinoma. European Journal of Cancer. 2013;**49**(16):3442-3449. DOI: 10.1016/j.ejca.2013.06.002

[61] Luo W, Hu H, Chang R, Zhong J, Knabel M, O'Meally R, et al. Pyruvate kinase M2 is a PHD3-stimulated coactivator for hypoxia-inducible factor 1. Cell. 2011;**145**(5):732-744. DOI: 10.1016/j.cell.2011.03.054

[62] Yang G, Zhang M, Zhao Y, Pan Y, Kan M, Li J, et al. HNF-4α inhibits hepatocellular carcinoma cell proliferation through mir-122-adam17 pathway. PLoS One. 2020;**15**(3):e0230450. DOI: 10.1371/journal.pone.0230450

[63] Jopling C. Liver-specific microRNA-122: Biogenesis and function. RNA Biology. 2012;**9**(2):137-142. DOI: 10.4161/rna.18827

[64] Coulouarn C, Factor VM, Andersen JB, Durkin ME, Thorgeirsson SS. Loss of miR-122 expression in liver cancer correlates with suppression of the hepatic phenotype and gain of metastatic properties. Oncogene. 2009;**28**(40):3526-3536. DOI: 10.1038/onc.2009.211

[65] Xiao G, Wang Q, Li B, Wu X, Liao H, Ren Y, et al. MicroRNA-338-3p Suppresses proliferation of human liver cancer cells by targeting SphK2. Oncology Research. 2018;**26**(8):1183-1189. DOI: 10.3727/096504018X15151495109394

[66] Wang B, Hsu SH, Frankel W, Ghoshal K, Jacob ST. Stat3-mediated activation of microRNA-23a suppresses gluconeogenesis in hepatocellular carcinoma by down-regulating glucose-6-phosphatase and peroxisome proliferator-activated receptor gamma, coactivator 1 alpha. Hepatology. 2012;**56**(1):186-197. DOI: 10.1002/hep.25632

[67] Mohamed AA, Ali-Eldin ZA, Elbedewy TA, El-Serafy M, Ali-Eldin FA, AbdelAziz H. MicroRNAs and clinical implications in hepatocellular carcinoma. World Journal of Hepatology. 2017;**9**(23):1001-1007. DOI: 10.4254/wjh.v9.i23.1001

[68] Zhu H, Han C, Wu T. MiR-17-92 cluster promotes hepatocarcinogenesis. Carcinogenesis. 2015;**36**(10):1213-1222. DOI: 10.1093/carcin/bgv112

[69] Mohr R, Özdirik B, Lambrecht J, et al. From liver cirrhosis to cancer: The role of micro-RNAs in hepatocarcinogenesis. International Journal of Molecular

Sciences. 2021;**22**(3):1492. DOI: 10.3390/ijms22031492

[70] Gao B, Gao K, Li L, Huang Z, Lin L. miR-184 functions as an oncogenic regulator in hepatocellular carcinoma (HCC). Biomedicine & Pharmacotherapy. 2014;**68**(2):143-148. DOI: 10.1016/j.biopha.2013.09.005

[71] Yang L, Peng F, Qin J, Zhou H, Wang B. Downregulation of microRNA-196a inhibits human liver cancer cell proliferation and invasion by targeting FOXO1. Oncology Reports. 2017;**38**(4):2148-2154. DOI: 10.3892/or.2017.5873

[72] Li X, Yuan M, Song L, Wang Y. Silencing of microRNA-210 inhibits the progression of liver cancer and hepatitis B virus-associated liver cancer via targeting EGR3. BMC Medical Genetics. 2020;**21**(1):48. DOI: 10.1186/s12881-020-0974-9

[73] Kim YC, Jung H, Seok S, et al. MicroRNA-210 promotes bile acid-induced cholestatic liver injury by targeting mixed-lineage leukemia-4 methyltransferase in mice. Hepatology. 2020;**71**(6):2118-2134. DOI: 10.1002/hep.30966

[74] Yang CL, Zheng XL, Ye K, et al. Effects of microRNA-217 on proliferation, apoptosis, and autophagy of hepatocytes in rat models of CCL4-induced liver injury by targeting NAT2. Journal of Cellular Physiology. 2019;**234**(4):3410-3424. DOI: 10.1002/jcp.26748

[75] Chen C, Matye D, Wang Y, Li T. Liver-specific microRNA-185 knockout promotes cholesterol dysregulation in mice. Liver Research. 2021;**5**(4):232-238

[76] Wang XC, Zhan XR, Li XY, Yu JJ, Liu XM. MicroRNA-185 regulates expression of lipid metabolism genes and improves insulin sensitivity in mice with non-alcoholic fatty liver disease. World Journal of Gastroenterology. 2014;**20**(47):17914-17923. DOI: 10.3748/wjg.v20.i47.17914

[77] Szabo G, Bala S. MicroRNAs in liver disease. Nature Reviews. Gastroenterology & Hepatology. 2013;**10**:542-552. DOI: 10.1038/nrgastro.2013.87

[78] Xie KL, Zhang YG, Liu J, Zeng Y, Wu H. MicroRNAs associated with HBV infection and HBV-related HCC. Theranostics. 2014;**4**:1176-1192. DOI: 10.7150/thno.8715

[79] Su C, Hou Z, Zhang C, Tian Z, Zhang J. Ectopic expression of microRNA-155 enhances innate antiviral immunity against HBV infection in human hepatoma cells. Virology Journal. 2011;**8**:354. DOI: 10.1186/1743-422X-8-354

[80] Yamada H, Suzuki K, Ichino N, Ando Y, Sawada A, Osakabe K, et al. Associations between circulating microRNAs (miR-21, miR-34a, miR-122 and miR-451) and non-alcoholic fatty liver. Clinica Chimica Acta. 2013;**424**:99-103. DOI: 10.1016/j.cca.2013.05.021

[81] McDaniel K, Huang L, Sato K, Wu N, Annable T, Zhou T, et al. The let-7/Lin28 axis regulates activation of hepatic stellate cells in alcoholic liver injury. The Journal of Biological Chemistry. 2017;**292**(27):11336-11347. DOI: 10.1074/jbc.M116.773291

[82] Wan Y, McDaniel K, Wu N, Ramos-Lorenzo S, Glaser T, Venter J, et al. Regulation of cellular senescence by miR-34a in alcoholic liver injury. The American Journal of Pathology. 2017;**187**(12):2788-2798. DOI: 10.1016/j.ajpath.2017.08.027

[83] Salvoza NC, Klinzing DC, Gopez-Cervantes J, Baclig MO. Association of circulating serum miR-34a and miR-122 with dyslipidemia among patients with non-alcoholic fatty liver disease. PLoS One. 2016;**11**(4):e0153497. DOI: 10.1371/journal.pone.0153497

[84] Li X, Zhang W, Xu K, Lu J. miR-34a promotes liver fibrosis in patients with chronic hepatitis via mediating Sirt1/p53 signaling pathway. Pathology, Research and Practice. 2020;**216**(5):152876. DOI: 10.1016/j.prp.2020.152876

[85] Zhang HF, Wang YC, Han YD. MicroRNA-34a inhibits liver cancer cell growth by reprogramming glucose metabolism. Molecular Medicine Reports. 2018;**17**(3):4483-4489. DOI: 10.3892/mmr.2018.8399

[86] Fornari F, Gramantieri L, Giovannini C, et al. MiR-122/cyclin G1 interaction modulates p53 activity and affects doxorubicin sensitivity of human hepatocarcinoma cells. Cancer Research. 2009;**69**(14):5761-5767. DOI: 10.1158/0008-5472.CAN-08-4797

[87] Momen-Heravi F, Catalano D, Talis A, Szabo G, Bala S. Protective effect of LNA-anti-miR-132 therapy on liver fibrosis in mice. Molecular Therapy--Nucleic Acids. 2021;**25**:155-167. DOI: 10.1016/j.omtn.2021.05.007

[88] Davis BN, Hilyard AC, Nguyen PH, Lagna G, Hata A. Smad proteins bind a conserved RNA sequence to promote microRNA maturation by Drosha. Molecular Cell. 2010;**39**(3):373-384. DOI: 10.1016/j.molcel.2010.07.011

[89] Chen S, Zhang J, Chen Q, Cheng J, Chen X, Mao Y, et al. MicroRNA-200a and microRNA-141 have a synergetic effect on the suppression of epithelial-mesenchymal transition in liver cancer by targeting STAT4. Oncology Letters. 2021;**21**(2):137. DOI: 10.3892/ol.2020.12398

[90] Dhayat SA, Mardin WA, Köhler G, Bahde R, Vowinkel T, Wolters H, et al. The microRNA-200 family--a potential diagnostic marker in hepatocellular carcinoma? Journal of Surgical Oncology. 2014;**110**(4):430-438. DOI: 10.1002/jso.23668

[91] Qin X, Zhang J, Lin Y, Sun XM, Zhang JN, Cheng ZQ. Identification of MiR-211-5p as a tumor suppressor by targeting ACSL4 in Hepatocellular Carcinoma. Journal of Translational Medicine. 2020;**18**(1):326. DOI: 10.1186/s12967-020-02494-7

[92] Jiang G, Cui Y, Yu X, Wu Z, Ding G, Cao L. miR-211 suppresses hepatocellular carcinoma by downregulating SATB2. Oncotarget. 2015;**6**(11):9457-9466. DOI: 10.18632/oncotarget.3265

[93] Cao MQ, You AB, Zhu XD, Zhang W, Zhang YY, Zhang SZ, et al. miR-182-5p promotes hepatocellular carcinoma progression by repressing FOXO3a. Journal of Hematology & Oncology. 2018;**11**(1):12. DOI: 10.1186/s13045-018-0555-y

[94] Yerukala-Sathipati S, Ho SY. Novel miRNA signature for predicting the stage of hepatocellular carcinoma. Scientific Reports. 2020;**10**(1):14452. DOI: 10.1038/s41598-020-71324-z

[95] Lu C, Liao Z, Cai M, Zhang G. MicroRNA-320a downregulation mediates human liver cancer cell proliferation through the Wnt/β-catenin signaling pathway. Oncology Letters. 2017;**13**(2):573-578. DOI: 10.3892/ol.2016.5479

[96] Wu L, Yang F, Lin B, et al. MicroRNA-424 expression predicts

tumor recurrence in patients with hepatocellular carcinoma following liver transplantation. Oncology Letters. 2018;**15**(6):9126-9132. DOI: 10.3892/ol.2018.8539

[97] Zha Z, Jia F, Hu P, Mai E, Lei T. MicroRNA-574-3p inhibits the malignant behavior of liver cancer cells by targeting ADAM28. Oncology Letters. 2020;**20**(3):3015-3023. DOI: 10.3892/ol.2020.11852

[98] Gao HB, Gao FZ, Chen XF. MiRNA-1179 suppresses the metastasis of hepatocellular carcinoma by interacting with ZEB2. European Review for Medical and Pharmacological Sciences. 2019;**23**(12):5149-5157. DOI: 10.26355/eurrev_201906_18179

[99] Tian Q, Liang L, Ding J, et al. MicroRNA-550a acts as a pro-metastatic gene and directly targets cytoplasmic polyadenylation element-binding protein 4 in hepatocellular carcinoma. PLoS One. 2012;**7**(11):e48958. DOI: 10.1371/journal.pone.0048958

[100] Rui T, Zhang X, Feng S, et al. The similar effects of miR-512-3p and miR-519a-2-5p on the promotion of hepatocellular carcinoma: Different Tunes Sung with equal skill. Frontiers in Oncology. 2020;**10**:1244

Chapter 6

Emerging Immunotherapy: Liver Cancer Microenvironment for Treatment

Shihai Liu

Abstract

Hepatocellular carcinoma (HCC) is a highly prevalent primary liver carcinoma and the main cause of deaths (linked with cancer) across the globe. Despite advancements in prevention strategies, testing, and technological advances in diagnosis and treatment, the occurrence and fatality rate of HCC continue to rise. In recent decades, the approval of immune checkpoint inhibitors (ICIs) has transformed palliative treatment for liver cancer. However, the majority of patients with liver cancer do not respond to these treatments. Herein, we elaborated the microenvironment of the liver cancer and candidate immunotherapies based on activating the antitumor activity of myeloid, NK and T cells, chimeric antigen receptors-T or -NK cells, vaccines, oncolytic viruses, and combination therapies, as well as the challenges and opportunities of immunotherapies in liver cancer. This review also explores the rationale, molecular foundation, and supporting preclinical evidence for immunotherapies in HCC, available clinical evidence, and current immunotherapeutic clinical studies.

Keywords: hepatocellular carcinoma, tumor-immune microenvironment, locoregional treatment, liver cirrhosis, systemic treatment

1. Introduction

Hepatocellular carcinoma (HCC) is the prevalent primary liver carcinoma and the largest cause of cancer-associated deaths across the globe. HCC accounts for ~90% of cases. Hepatitis B and C virus infections, liver flukes in endemic areas, excessive intake of alcohol, cigarettes, elevated level of body fat, and aflatoxins are all significant risk factors for developing HCC. The tumor burden, liver functioning, comorbidities, and health condition of a patient influence treatment options for HCC. HCC treatments have changed dramatically over the past four decades. Surgical or organ transplantation is the first-line treatment for tumors less than 5 cm in diameter. However, the treatment of large HCCs (those greater than 10 cm) is disputed, with considerable heterogeneity in various treatment regimens in different locations [1]. Additionally, radiofrequency ablation (RFA) and transarterial chemoembolization (TACE) are the local modalities utilized for early and intermediate-stage HCC, accordingly [2, 3]. Systemic treatments for advanced-stage HCC were found controversial prior to 2008 because of their ineffectiveness and poor patient tolerability. Moreover, systemic treatments for liver cancers have made little progress in the last decade.

Immuno-oncology has revolutionized cancer treatment, particularly liver cancer, over the last decade. The antitumor immune response combines innate and adaptive immune system elements [4]. Tumors, on the other hand, can harness this response and use it to evade the immune system in a variety of ways, including maintaining an immunosuppressive milieu or inducing cytotoxic cell malfunctions. An immunosuppressive tumor immune microenvironment (TIME) is marked by the existence of regulatory T cells (Treg), immunosuppressive myeloid cells including tumor-associated macrophages (TAMs), and inhibitory B cells [5]. Immune checkpoint activation, which includes coinhibitory substances, prevents effector cell activation and is crucial for tumor immune evasion [6]. Cancer treatment has been transformed by the development of immune checkpoint inhibitor (ICI)-based therapy, which has led to long-term responses and improved survival in a wide spectrum of cancers. However, ICIs have not been very effective against many solid tumors. Checkpoint proteins expressed by immune cells or tumor cells serve as targets for ICI monoclonal antibodies (mAbs), which elicit a robust immunological response from cytotoxic T lymphocytes (CTLs) [7]. Moreover, ICI therapy has shown to be effective in a subset of patients with a range of cancers, including HCC. Anti-PDL1 antibody atezolizumab and the VEGF neutralizing antibody bevacizumab are now the standard therapies for HCC [8]. Herein, we explored the rationale, molecular basis, and underlying preclinical evidence for immunotherapies in HCC, along with existing immunological clinical research.

2. Overview of immune components

2.1 Immune cells

The liver is a key immunological organ that receives antigen-rich blood from the gut via the portal vein. Cancer immunosurveillance and control rely heavily on the innate and adaptive immune systems. The conflicting actions of antitumor effectors and their suppressors in the TME determine immune activation or evasion, as shown in (**Figure 1**). Through highly conserved cytokine and chemokine-activated inflammatory reactions, adaptive and innate immune cells patrol the liver sinusoids to eliminate invading pathogens and endotoxins. The uninflamed liver generates a

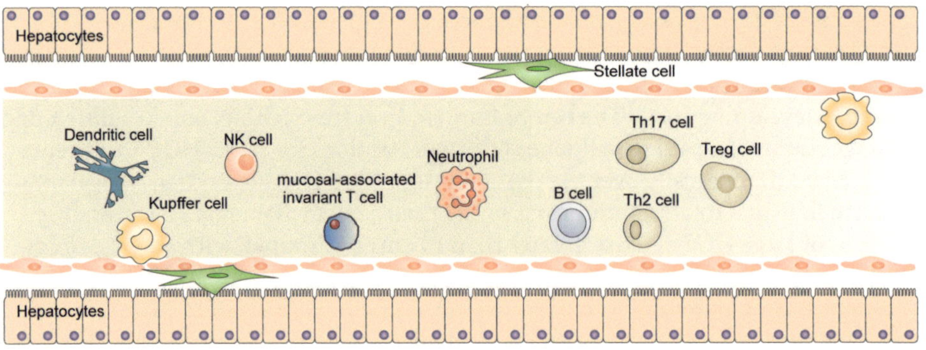

Figure 1.
Homeostasis and immune cell composition of the liver.

tolerogenic milieu that suppresses both innate and adaptive immunity in order to maintain homeostasis and prevent chronic inflammation and tissue damage. The immune cell composition of the TME has a huge impact on HCC that can affect tumor initiation, progression, and therapeutic response. During hepatocarcinogenesis, several molecular processes cause distinct immune cell subsets to respond in ways that either cause inflammation or limit antitumor immunity. Herein, the immune cell landscape of HCC is discussed, with an emphasis on the role of innate immune cells and innate-like T cells in HCC, which may lead to the development of candidate immunotherapies that target the underlined cells.

2.2 Cytokines

HCC's genesis and progression have been linked to inflammation. TNF-α, a key inflammatory mediator, had previously been identified as a possible therapeutic target in a variety of malignancies. Furthermore, TNF-α, interleukin (IL)-1, and IL-6 levels in HCC patients' serum were found to be considerably greater than in healthy controls. CXCL5 and CCL15, which are produced by tumor cells, attract immunosuppressive neutrophils and monocytes, respectively, while CXCL13, which is produced by hepatic stellate cells, attracts B cells, which differentiate into protumor IgA-producing plasma cells in the context of NASH-associated HCC. IL-2, IFNγ, CXCL10, and CXCL9, on the other hand, recruit lymphocytes to mount an antitumor immune reaction. As a result, the immunological composition and response are determined by the balance of these stimuli. T helper 17 (Th17) cells generate the cytokine IL-17, which has been linked to the development and progression of inflammatory disorders. These findings have ramifications for patients who are undergoing immunotherapy. Activation of the IFN-γ signaling system predicts a favorable response to ICIs, according to the findings of two trials in patients with HCC. In HCC, the tumor microenvironment (TME) has a significant impact on cytokine production.

2.3 Signaling cascades lead to immune evasion

HCC's immune microenvironment can be influenced by tumor intrinsic signaling pathways. Wnt ligands produced by HCC cells induce M2 polarization of TAMs, which results in tumor development, metastasis, and immunosuppression in HCC. β-Catenin signaling also inhibits MHC-independent immune responses facilitated by NK cells through decreased expression of NKG2D ligands on HCC cells. By reversing NK cell depletion or TGF- β1 reversing NK cell depletion, blocking the CD96 association restores NK cell immunity to tumors, implying that CD96 may considerably contribute to HCC. MYC may suppress PD-L1 expression in HCC, which suggested that treating HCC with a combination therapy targeting MYC and the PD-L1/PD-1 cascade could be beneficial. HCC is linked to TP53 gene mutations and immune cell heterogeneity, with TP53 mutations reported in roughly 40% of all HCCs. The TP53 mutation-associated immunotype is critical for better clinical outcomes and may have important implications for postoperative tailored follow-up and therapeutic decision-making. Furthermore, ARID1A mutations, which are a common driving factor in HCC, have a considerable contribution to antitumor immunity: they stimulate a positive response by suppressing mismatch repair, leading to an elevated TMB, and also reduce IFNγ signaling by lowering chromatin availability. In co-cultured CD4+ T cells, MDSC suppresses the immune system by generating CD4+ CD25+ Foxp3+ regulatory T cells. The IL6-STAT3-PDL1 signaling cascade is used by HCC-CAFs to control neutrophil survival, stimulation, and function in HCC. Finally, T cell fatigue is caused by the upregulation of immunological checkpoint molecules such as PD-1, PDL1, CTLA4, LAG3, and TIM3 in HCC cells. PDL1 overexpression in Kupffer cells and leukocytes is also caused by prolonged HBV infection, which can boost the protein's level and enhance immunosuppression in HCCs of this etiology.

2.4 Virus associated with HCC

HCC is the main cause of death in cirrhotic patients, with HCV or HBV infection accounting for the majority of cases, especially in developing countries. HBV is a hepatotropic virus that causes liver inflammation. While another established risk factor for severe liver disease is HCV, a Flaviviridae virus. Long-term infection with HBV or HCV causes an inflammatory reaction in the liver that can develop into cirrhosis and, ultimately, HCC.

HBV and HCV-induced immune responses might be either procarcinogenic or anticarcinogenic. Platelets generate components that induce a necroinflammatory infiltration, *i.e.,* virus-specific CD8 + T cells, which drive HCC development and can be slowed down with antiplatelet medications. An effective HBV-specific T cell response, on the other hand, can aid in the control of HCC cells displaying HBV epitopes, as clinically demonstrated by tumor regressions accomplished with adoptive T cells genetically modified to produce TCRs targeting such epitopes. Despite this, persistent HBV infection causes multiple changes in the hepatic immune infiltrate, which promote a tolerogenic milieu, limiting effective antitumor immunity. B reg cells are a primary source of IL-10, an immunosuppressive cytokine that is increased during HBV flares. Furthermore, HBV-specific T cells are susceptible to BIM-induced apoptotic process and TRAIL + NKG2D + NK cell deletion. Chronic HBV infection also increases the production of inhibitory immunological checkpoint proteins on virus-specific T cells, mainly in the liver, restricting any T cells capable of attacking HCC cells. In patients with HBV-associated HCC, the presence of elevated suppressive PD-1 T reg cells is linked with worse survival outcomes, although CD8+ tissue-resident memory T cells are correlated with a better outcome.

HCV has a single polyprotein genome, which is translated into structural as well as nonstructural proteins. These HCV proteins are targets for the host's innate and adaptive immune systems. The principal pattern recognition receptors that identify HCV PAMPs are RIG-I-like receptors and Toll-like receptors. The correlation stimulates a cascade of antiviral cytokines, including interferons. Perforin, as well as granzyme B, is secreted by CD8 + T cells and NK cells while interferon-gamma (IFN-γ) secreted by CD8 + T cells and NK cells causes noncytolytic HCV clearance. Moreover, the host-HCV interactions could make developing an HCV vaccine challenging. It is hard to neutralize a virus that typically has so many mutations in its E1 and E2 proteins, and attempts to do so clear the most abundant variants and leave replicative space for the expansion and continued replication of other quasispecies.

Understanding how virus-related HCCs regulate their metabolism could open up new avenues for immunotherapy. By decreasing arginine, granulocytic MDSCs accumulate in HBV-infected livers and can suppress HBV-specific T cells. High expression of the esterification enzyme sterol Oacyltransferase 1 (SOAT1) disrupts lipid homeostasis, promoting proliferative and migratory potential of the tumor cell in a subset of HBV-associated HCCs while reducing the activity of HBV/HCC-specific tumor-infiltrating lymphocytes.

2.5 Nonviral HCC

Hepatic steatosis and chronic necroinflammation in the liver can result from persistent alcohol exposure or high-calorie diets combined with a sedentary lifestyle, leading to HCC, which could be fatal. Moreover, NASH-induced inflammation is more frequently linked with diffuse inflammatory infiltrates.

New developments regarding the cellular and molecular cascades that drive NASH and the NASH-HCC transition have emerged in recent years. It has been revealed that platelets drive NASH and the NASH-HCC transition by fostering the first inflammatory reactions in the context of steatosis. Platelets interact with Kupffer cells and inflammatory monocytes through the platelet-specific glycoprotein Ibα (GPIbα). In rodents, and possibly also in humans, preventive and therapeutic antiplatelet treatment lowers the development of NASH and NASH-associated HCC. The study revealed that the usage of low-dose aspirin is linked with a considerably decreased risk of HCC and liver-associated death. NASH-related liver cancer is caused by a variety of immunological mechanisms. NKT cells mediate lipid uptake via LTβR activation on hepatocytes, and metabolic stimulation of intrahepatic CD8 + T cells and NKT cells, for example, has been demonstrated to induce NASH and HCC via hepatocyte cross talk. NKT cells primarily cause steatosis via secreted LIGHT, while CD8+ and NKT cells cooperatively induce liver damage. The metabolic machinery in hepatocytes is downregulated as a result of this cross talk, which involves direct interaction between immune cells and hepatocytes via Fas and release of porforins and granzymes as well as indirect communication via secreted substances (e.g., cytokines, chemokines), resulting in increased metabolic, endoplasmic reticulum, and mitochondrial stress. Surprisingly, human NASH has been found to have a considerable elevation in the number of intrahepatic CD8 + PD1 + T cells. As previously stated, metabolic imbalance triggers autoaggression in these CD8 + PD1 + T cells, culminating in MHC I independent cytotoxicity against hepatocytes and necroinflammation. This autoaggressive behavior of CD8 + PD1 + T cells has implications for patients receiving ICIs for NASH-associated HCC: nonviral HCCs, particularly NASH-associated HCCs, are less susceptible to these drugs than viral HCCs. This discrepancy has been linked to the autoaggressive intratumoral CD8 + PD1 + T cells losing their tumor surveillance function, resulting in a protumorigenic milieu.

Alcohol consumption is responsible for up to 30% of all HCC cases worldwide. The mucosal damage caused by alcohol might result in an impaired intestinal barrier function, enabling toxins of gut-inhabiting bacteria such as endotoxins to enter the systemic circulation and to contribute to liver injury after alcohol consumption. Alcohol increases gut permeability, allowing immunomodulatory microbiota-derived PAMPs such as LPS to enter the liver and decrease hepatic immune reactions, presumably through effects on resident macrophages. NASH is linked to an increase in protumorigenic, immunosuppressive granulocytic MDSCs in the liver, as well as a decrease in T cell migration to the liver. Furthermore, the neutrophils in the liver parenchyma are a hallmark of alcoholic hepatitis, which is thought to influence the hepatic immune landscape.

2.6 The modulatory of the microbiota

Dysbiosis has been seen in various phases of chronic liver injury, including HCC, according to several investigations. The gut microbiota increases HCC development in the setting of chronic liver injury, presumably via microbial metabolites or PAMPs, according to in vivo studies using a mouse model. Through the primary to the secondary conversion of luminal bile acids, the microbiota of the stomach can reduce immunosurveillance and accelerate the progression of HCC. Furthermore, metabolized bile acids (deoxycholic acid, a secondary bile acid) have been demonstrated to cause senescence in hepatic stellate cells, leading to the production of numerous cytokines such as transforming growth factor-β1, angiotensin II, leptin) that enhance the progression of HCC. The relevance of the gut microbiota in influencing systemic immunity, including immunotherapeutic reactions and chemotherapy-induced immunological effects, is now widely recognized. The antigenic epitope tail length tape measure protein 1 (TMP1) in the genome of bacteriophage Enterococcus hirae had high similarity with the proteasome subunit beta type-4 (PSMB4) tumor antigen. They activated CD8+ T cells simultaneously and improved the efficacy of PD-1 blockade therapy. It has been demonstrated that the antigen epitope SVYRYYGL (SVY) expressed in the commensal bacterium Bifidobacterium breve was similar to the tumor-expressed antigen epitope SIYRYYGL (SIY), resulting in SVY-specific T cells recognizing SIY and inhibiting tumor growth. However, further research on the impacts on hepatic immunity is still needed.

2.7 HCC immune classification

Few studies have attempted to classify HCC according to its immunological status. The "Inflammatory" and "Lymphocyte Depleted" clusters were found prominent in HCCs, according to a pancancer analysis based on clustering of immune-associated gene expression profiles. Using a transcriptome deconvolution technique, the first thorough immune categorization of HCC was published in 2017, which found an "Immune" class (which accounts for 25% of HCCs). Immune tumors have an elevated level of immune infiltration, enhanced PD-1/PDL1 signaling, and signature enrichment that mimics the response to ICIs in other solid tumor types.

More recently, a modification of this classification established an "Inflamed" class of HCC, which accounts for about 30–35% of tumors, expanding the previously documented immune class with an additional subset of tumors labeled as an "Immune-like" subclass. This novel subclass is distinguished by the presence of CTNNB1 mutations and significant activation of interferon signaling and immunological activation. T-cell-inflamed tumors are characterized by type I interferon (IFN) activation, immune potentiating chemokines, antigen presentation, cytotoxic effector molecules, and activated CD8+ T cells. The inflamed tumor microenvironment is additionally characterized by IFN-induced inhibitory pathways such as programmed death-ligand 1 (PD-L1) and indoleamine-2, 3 dioxygenase and higher proportions of FOXP3+ regulatory T cells. Patients with HCC have a higher proportion of inflamed tumors, and those patients who responded to anti-PD-1/PDL1 antibodies were shown to be enriched in the inflamed class. In the "Noninflamed" class of HCCs, two subclasses have been evaluated based on the mechanisms of immune escape: (1) an "Intermediate" class with TP53 mutations, elevated levels of chromosomal instability, and frequent deletions in subcytobands harboring genes linked with interferon signaling or antigen presentation; and (2) an "Excluded" class with CTNNB1 mutations and immune desertification features.

3. Landscape of immunotherapy for HCC

3.1 Immunotherapy for early-stage HCC

Early-stage (BCLC 0 and BCLCA) HCC patients can benefit from treatments such as surgery, liver transplantation, and radiofrequency ablation (RFA) [9]. However, recurrence after liver surgery is prevalent and closely linked to poor overall survival, with recurrence rates of up to 50% and 70% following 2 and 5 years, accordingly [1]. Recurrence is linked to the manifestation of thrombocytopenia, cirrhosis, and satellite lesions [10]. Furthermore, various immunological variables were found with relatively poor resection effects. High PD-L1 expression is linked to an elevated level of immunosuppressive molecules including regulatory T-cells (also known as Tregs) and myeloid-derived suppressor cells (MDSCs) as well as the attenuation of cytotoxic elements such as interferonγ [11–14]. High CD3+ and CD8+ T cell density in the tumor core and margin, as well as related immune scores, which are based on the number of CD3+ and CD8+ lymphocytes in the intratumor (from the tumor core to the periphery), are linked to a much lower probability of HCC recurrence postsurgical treatment [15, 16]. For patients with unresectable HCC or HCC with end-stage liver disease, liver transplantation is an alternate and possibly ideal therapeutic option. However, only a small percentage of HCC patients match the transplant criteria, and the restricted number of transplant centers makes liver transplantation an unrealistic option for many patients due to the chronic shortage of donor organs. Hence, it is needed to combine adjuvant and neoadjuvant immunotherapy to elevate the likelihood of cure post HCC surgery.

3.1.1 Adjuvant treatment

Post resection, numerous adjuvant therapies were undertaken in the hopes of enhancing survival, but none of them was found successful. Systemic treatment has relied heavily on sorafenib over the previous decade, making it the only medicine approved for first-line treatment since 2017. Currently, the approval of lenvatinib has been accepted in the practice of first-line setting [17]. T lymphocytes that have been grown ex vivo with cytokines make up CIK cells. In an open-label, phase-3 trial involving 230 patients (associated with HCC) who experienced surgical resection, patients who got CIK lived 44 months longer than those who received placebo (HR, 0.63; 95% CI 0.43–0.94; $p = 0.010$). However, despite these recent advancements, no adjuvant therapy has consistently proven effective.

3.1.2 Neoadjuvant therapy

Neoadjuvant therapy is a treatment strategy applied prior to the primary cancer treatment to enhance the rate of success for the primary treatment. In neoadjuvant therapy, ICIs can take advantage of the elevated levels of tumor antigens present in the primary tumor to enhance the proliferative potential of tumor-specific T lymphocyte clones already existing in the TME [18]. Mice administered neoadjuvant Tregs level was reduced due to diphtheria toxin fragments. While anti-CD25 lived considerably longer (250 days) than control mice (100 days) in preclinical models of triple-negative breast cancer [19]. A limited time interval between the first administration of neoadjuvant immunotherapy and primary tumor excision was found essential for maximum efficacy in a second trial, whereas a greater time interval abolished therapeutic efficacy in the neoadjuvant context. The viability of neoadjuvant cabozantinib with nivolumab in HCC was investigated in a single-arm phase 1b study [18]. The trial included 15 unresectable patients, 12 of whom had successful margin-negative resection after neoadjuvant cabozantinib and nivolumab therapy. Furthermore, responders showed enrichment of CD138+ plasma cells and a specific spatial rearrangement of B cells, with B cells in close proximity to other B cells, indicating that this combination modulated the TIME. These findings point to the need for a B-cell orchestration of antitumor immune responses. Immunotherapy is also being researched as a neoadjuvant treatment for liver transplantation. In HCC patients that meet the Milan criteria, the combination of lenvatinib and pembrolizumab is being tested in PLENTY202001 before liver transplantation. The usage of ICIs in the transplant scenario poses considerable safety concerns, as it can result in allograft rejection, which can be deadly [20]. As a result, solid organ patients are routinely excluded from clinical trials employing ICIs. The PLENTY202001 is an outlier in this regard, as it will collect extremely valuable safety data.

3.2 Intermediate HCC immunotherapy

TACE is the gold standard of therapy for intermediate-stage BCLC-HCC (B). This immunotherapy significantly improves OS [21]. In addition, TACE seems to influence the immunological response of tumors [22–24]. TACE can improve both the antitumor immune response and the pro-inflammatory tumor response by lowering Tregs and fatigued effector T-cells in the tumor core [23]. HCC patients (n = 32) who were not eligible for liver surgical resection or transplantation were evaluated for the efficacy and safety of tremelimumab (anti-CTLA-4) with ablation [25]. Tremelimumab was given to patients every 4 weeks for six doses. They had TACE (subtotal radiofrequency ablation) on day 36. Five of the 19 evaluable patients had an established partial response, and the median OS was 19.4 months. Six-week tumor biopsies revealed an increase in CD8+ T cells in those individuals who had a therapeutic benefit. Hence, the combination of locoregional plus immunotherapy for HCC at the intermediate stage is mechanistically justified. Because it enrolled patients with unresectable HCC. Furthermore, The IMbrave 150 trial revealed information regarding HCC-associated patients at an intermediate stage [8]. The ABC-HCC study proposes a novel type of primary endpoint called time-to-failure of treatment strategy, which assesses the time until the investigator discontinues either treatment strategy (systemic therapy or TACE) due to failure [26].

3.3 Immunotherapy for advanced-stage HCC

Immunotherapy has been shown to be effective in the treatment of advanced HCC. ICIs, particularly those that target PD-1 or PD-L1, are the most commonly used drugs. They've been studied in big clinical studies both individually and in combination, and they have now become an important aspect of HCC treatment. Furthermore, new immunotherapies, including adoptive cell therapy with considerable improvement in ICI's therapeutic efficacy against HCC.

3.3.1 Monotherapies with ICIs

A monoclonal antibody, *i.e.,* nivolumab, targeting PD-1, was originally investigated in HCC in phase I/II CheckMate 040 investigation, which comprised 262 HCC patients with a previous history of sorafenib treatment. Nivolumab had a median response length of 73.87 weeks (95% confidence interval (CI) 6–24) and an ORR of 14 percent by RECIST 1.1 (18% by mRECIST) [27]. The study found a median OS of 15.6 months and a safety profile that was similar to prior nivolumab trials. As a result, the FDA granted nivolumab expedited approval for patients with advanced-stage HCC who had previously received sorafenib treatment. In the CheckMate 459 research, nivolumab was compared with sorafenib as a first-line treatment in patients with advanced HCC who had not previously undergone systemic treatment.

In HCC patients (with a previous history of sorafenib treatment) after intolerable toxicity or rejection of sorafenib, the trial-22 (phase 1/2) found a median OS of 65.6 months (95% CI 7.7–24.6) and a median PFS of 8.69 months (95% CI 1.8–5.4) with an acceptable safety profile for tremelimumab monotherapy. Tremelimumab plus durvalumab (anti-PD-L1), on the other hand, had a better overall benefit–risk ratio [28]. Furthermore, early growth of Ki67+ CD8 + T cells was linked to response to either the single treatment or the combination. This is the final trial that potentially leads to global regulatory clearance for a single drug checkpoint inhibitor. The focus and expectations have shifted to combination therapies in general.

3.3.2 Dual therapeutic strategy using ICIs and anti-VEGF antibodies

Based on the positive results of the IMbrave150 phase-3 trial 8, the combination of a PD1/PD-L1 inhibitor and a VEGF blocker has become a new strategy to treat advanced HCC [8]. The IMbrave150 experiment resulted in the approval of atezolizumab plus bevacizumab as first-line treatment for unresectable HCC in the United States and Europe, replacing the TKIs sorafenib and lenvatinib. Inhibition of PD-L1, which increases the immune response (especially T-effector cells), and inhibition of VEGF, which stimulates T-cell infiltration in the tumor microenvironment and overcomes VEGF-mediated immunosuppression, is thought to have synergistic antitumor efficacy [29].

The ORIENT-32 phase 2/3 trial compared sintilimab (anti-PD1) and IBI305 (a bevacizumab biosimilar) to sorafenib in systemic treatment-naive Chinese patients, similar to the IMbrave150 trial (NCT03794440). In comparison to sorafenib, sintilimab/IBI305 exhibited an elevated median OS and PFS (median OS: not attained vs. 10.4 months; median PFS: 41.2 weeks vs. 12.17 weeks) with acceptable tolerability of [30].

3.3.3 Combination therapies of PD-1 and CTLA-4 inhibitors

Immune checkpoint inhibitor therapy for cancer patients has undoubtedly been a big achievement in oncology in recent years, and it represents a huge stride forward as a novel type of immunotherapy in cancer treatment. The combined ICIs including (anti-CTLA-4, and anti-PD-1/L1) are currently being investigated in advanced HCC. The CheckMate 040 trial, which evaluated nivolumab with ipilimumab in 148 patients with advanced HCC who had developed resistance to sorafenib, yielded the first clinical data [31]. The underlined therapy has been approved by the FDA post successful results of the trials. Moreover, systemic steroids are needed to treat adverse events.

3.3.4 Combination therapies of the checkpoint and multi-kinase inhibitors

Anti-VEGF antibodies can be replaced with ICIs and TKIs to inhibit VEGF. Currently, several such combinations are being investigated. As a secondary outcome measure, cabinozantinib monotherapy is compared with sorafenib. In a phase 1b trial involving 104 patients with unresectable HCC, the combination of lenvatinib with pembrolizumab was found to have potential anticancer efficacy [32].

Finally, camrelizumab (SHR1210, anti-PD-1) and apatinib (rivoceranib, a TKI inhibits VEGFR2) were tested in the clinic. An ORR of 50% was observed in a phase 1 investigation of individuals with advanced HCC [33]. The combination therapies are being evaluated as a first-line treatment for patients with advanced HCC in the phase 3 clinical trial.

3.3.5 Systemic treatment beyond ICIs

The most common method of cancer immunotherapy is the attenuation of the immunological checkpoints PD1/PD-L1 and CTLA-4. LAG-3 is an alternative immunological checkpoint that suppresses T-cell function, indicating T-cell depletion. In phase 2 RELATIVITY-073 trial in advanced, ICI-naive HCC post-progression on prior TKI therapy, relatlimab, an antibody that blocks LAG-3, is being tested in combination with nivolumab. Additionally, a growing number of novel immunotherapeutic methods are being investigated. Where today's ICIs fail, such interventions could be effective. Adoptive transfer of NK or T cells to increase tumor infiltration, for example, could benefit patients whose tumors aren't infiltrated by effector immune cells.

Besides classic checkpoint inhibition, the majority of immunotherapies are still in the preclinical or early clinical stages, and these include allogeneic NK cells, CAR-T, as well as oncolytic viruses [34]. CAR-T cells targeting GPC3 are currently being studied in phase 1 trials. Moreover, autologous T cells expressing improved TCRs specific for AFP (AFP c332 T) are being tested in HLA-A2-positive people with advanced HCC in the first phase 1 experiment targeting AFP. Pexastimogene devacirepvec (Pexa-Vec) failed in the TRAVERSE phase 2b trial and the PHOCUS trial as a second-line monotherapy in advanced HCC [35, 36]. Pexa-Vec and nivolumab are currently being tested in a phase 1/2a experiment. Novel immunotherapeutic techniques have the potential to provide immunotherapy benefits to a larger number of patients. However, it is not yet obvious which approaches will enhance or even replace current systemic therapeutic strategies.

4. Other HCC immunotherapies

4.1 Adoptive cell therapy (ACT)

In ACT combined with effector cells, lymphocytes are activated and/or amplified ex vivo before being reintroduced into the patients. Redirected peripheral blood T cells, TILs, CIK cells, NK cells, and lymphokine-activated killer cells (LAKs) are among the cell types that are used in this procedure. T-lymphocytes in the peripheral circulation have been genetically recoded to preferentially target tumor cells. The two basic techniques are chimeric antigen receptors (CARs) and transgenic tumor antigen-specific TCRs. CIK, TIL, and LAK therapies are not affected by the cancer-associated genes. Except in LAK, CIK, and CAR T cells, MHC-specific antitumor activity has been found in TIL and TCR-redirected cells. Usually, adoptive transplant cells are preconditioned with fludarabine and cyclophosphamide to promote lymphodepletion and enhance in vivo growth. Patients receiving LAK, CIK, or TIL treatment are often given IL-2 to assist the transferred cells' proliferation in vivo.

Because of the technology's apparent complexity and absence of efficiency, the first attempts to use ACT to treat HCC never got to the clinical stage. The fact that LAK cells poorly develop ex-vivo and have a poor cytolytic impact in melanoma patients serves as an example of the intricacy of this system. HCC recurrence was reduced by using LAK cells as an additive following resection to reduce the risk of HCC recurrence. However, this had not improved survival. However, CIK cells are more cytotoxic and proliferative when compared with LAK cells. NKT cells principally contribute to the antitumor effect of this diverse population. In 2015, a multicenter, randomized phase III trial involving 226 patients demonstrated that combination immunotherapy with CIK cells increased PFS and OS of HCC patients following percutaneous ablation or curative surgical resection relative to the patients who did not receive combination therapy. Considering the underlined outcomes, the majority of institutions do not use ACT as adjuvant therapy, most likely due to a lack of in-house cell therapy facilities. From tumor samples (fresh), TILs were obtained followed by selecting the tumor-reactive growing cells on the basis of their autologous cell recognition. Next, these cells were amplified to produce many active cells. The effectiveness of combined TIL treatment was indicated in a Phase-I study with individuals who had HCC7. TILs were given to 15 of 17 patients, with doses up to 3 × 10 [9] cells administered with the least side effects. The major challenges for clinical usage are obtaining sufficient T-cells that are selective for tumor neoepitopes and shortening the underlined procedure.

NK cells have a wide spectrum of receptors that allow them to identify tumor cells even without prior sensitization or the acquisition of receptor reconfiguration. For clinical usage, their inability to grow in vitro may be overcome. Phase II clinical trials are now using allogeneic NK cells to treat patients who have an increased risk of HCC recurrence following surgery or TACE.

In the treatment of hematologic malignancies (such as leukemia, multiple myeloma, and lymphoma), CAR T cell therapy has shown significant promise; however, its use in solid tumors is still under investigation. CAR T cells express transmembrane, intracellular signaling domains, and antigen-recognition domains that are common features of CAR T cells. One-chain variable fragments produced from the variable heavy and light chains of monoclonal antibodies selective for certain tumor cell targets, which can be tumor antigens, usually make up the extracellular antigen-recognition domains. In HCC, GPC3 has emerged as the most specific and appealing target. The efficacy of orthotopic and patient-derived xenografts has been demonstrated in various animal models. One of the most serious issues with CAR T cells is off-target toxicity. This occurs when the expression of the targeting molecule is in non-tumor tissues.

According to several studies, AFP is often overexpressed in HCC. Due to its intracellular expression and secretion, TCR-based therapy is relatively more effective when compared with CAR-based therapies. In patients associated with HCC, four HLA-A2-restricted AFP epitopes were identified. TP53 hotspot mutations, which are common in HCC and HBV antigens, are two more possible targets for T-cells (TCR-engineered).

4.2 Therapeutic vaccines

The key stimulus for using cancer vaccines is to induce tumor-specific reactions with higher efficacy. The underlined impact can be obtained by de novo priming T-cells against antigens produced by tumor cells that do not generate a spontaneous response and further enhancing the remaining reactions or expanding the repertoire and breadth of tumor-specific responses. Vaccinations were once thought to be a stand-alone treatment. However, it is now obvious that they should be used in combination with ICIs or ACT. Combinations of ICIs could block these variables, making it easier for antitumor lymphocytes to accomplish their activities.

In situ therapeutic vaccines act by activating tumor-infiltrating APCs, which absorb and display endogenous TAAs. Classic tumor vaccines, on the other hand, rely on the exogenous delivery of antigens or antigen-pulsed DCs. Cancer antigens should be immunogenic enough to overcome the tolerance induced by multiple self-molecules appearing on tumor cells, while also conferring selectivity for tumor cells and blocking the response of non-tumor cells. Antigen identity is uncertain in tumor lysate, which comprises self-molecules that could not confirm the accurate view of relevant TAA. Using tumor cell lysates as a treatment for HCC in a number of trials did not lead to consistent results.

TAAs including GPC-3, AFP, and telomerase have been addressed as HCC peptide vaccines (antigens specific). HCC patients have revealed spontaneous T-cell responses to the above antigens, suggesting that they are immunogenic in some way. In the majority of cases, T-cell sensitivity to their corresponding antigen is unclear. Hardly a few telomerase and GPC-3-targeting techniques have progressed to clinical evaluations, and none of them has yielded clinically relevant data that could serve as an active pharmaceutical candidate. One of the problems with the approach of therapeutic vaccination is tumor phenotypic heterogeneity and the real possibility that despite best efforts, some tumor cells will simply not be targeted by the vaccine, even if the vaccine is multivalent.

The identification of real tumor-specific antigens should be used to develop more immunogenic vaccinations. HLA peptidomics approaches are the first option that can be used to identify peptides that utilize peptides and serve as a unique immunological signature that CTLs may identify. On the basis of this method, a vaccine clinical evaluation has completed recruitment in HCC.

The use of neoantigens is a second approach. Their detection is based on a complicated pathway that involves analyzing mutations in tumor cells in comparison with wild-type cells. This method is utilized to investigate mutant gene expression as well as immune-associated factors including epitope process ability and HLA molecule interaction. Furthermore, the method has been used to anticipate significantly immunogenic neoantigens with antitumor potential as vaccines in different tumors, including glioblastoma and melanoma. There is a need for extensive studies to clinically evaluate HCC. Only a limited number of studies have been reported that relate the existence of mutations to specific immune responses. According to the results obtained from our ongoing research, mutations observed in HCC patients may generate peptides with stronger HLA-interacting potential when compared with non-mutated wild-type sequences. This research is still being conducted by our group. It has been shown that these peptides stimulate T-cells to recognize only the mutant sequence and not the wild type in HLA-transgenic mice, implying that the method could possibly be used as a vaccination for HCC.

5. Locoregional therapies

The immune system has developed to deal with microbial infections as well as severe tissue injuries. These situations are recognized by interconnected innate receptors, the function of which determines whether or not an adaptive immune response is produced and progresses. Furthermore, these activities may influence whether tumor antigens trigger immunization, tolerance, or not. As a result, hard efforts have been made over the years in order to develop cancerous tissue that seems like diseased or stressed tissue, which might encourage cytotoxic immunity's adaptive response. Immune cell death and the use of PAMPs are two important concepts to look into in this context.

Immunogenic cell death (ICD) occurs when cells secrete or synthesize alarmins, a group of proteins that signal and stimulate APCs, i.e., DCs. ICD is linked to ER stress, necroptosis or necrosis, the secretion of mitochondrial and nuclear substances, and the activation of the Type-I IFNs. Moreover, chemo and radiotherapies, as well as other physical stimuli, activate cell and tissue damage and enhance immunity against tumor progression.

The immune system is activated by entities other than viruses, bacteria, and other prokaryotic entities. This reactivity allows drugs such as inflammasome agonists, Toll-like receptor (TLR) agonists, MDA5 or RIGI agonists, and cGAS–STING agonists to be delivered locally, stimulating localized immunity. These substances are usually synthetic analogs or obtained from microbial products, and when administered systemically, cause systemic inflammation and sepsis-like cytokine secretion syndromes. They may be more potent in triggering an immunological response with fewer adverse effects when administered intratumorally. Microorganisms can boost antitumor immunity without using their immune-stimulating substances. Therefore, Bacillus Calmette-Guérin vaccine is used for the local treatment of superficial bladder carcinoma. Oncolytic virotherapy is an effective therapeutic technique against cancer progression. This technique employs viruses that proliferate specifically in cancerous cells in order to kill them, with promising results in HCC. But instead of the cytopathic effects of the viruses, it has become clear that most of the therapeutic benefits of virotherapy come from boosting immune responses that target tumor antigens. Also, spores of anerobic bacteria have been used to amplify immune responses against tumors, since they only germinate in hypoxic environments, which occur in tumor nodules. This is why some bacterial infections trigger immune stimulation that in turn target tumor cells.

Locoregional methods are highly recommended for the treatment of individuals with unresectable HCC. Catheter-based procedures (yttrium-90 irradiation and transarterial chemoembolization) and locoregional ablative treatments, either chemical (percutaneous ethanol injection) or thermal (thermal ablation), are examples of image-guided therapies (laser, microwave, and radiofrequency ablation, and cryoablation) [4]. HCC is favorable for local therapies that can trigger ICD or local delivery of PAMPs due to its easy availability to tumor-affected regions. Notably, multiple locoregional therapies can be used independently or in combination with systemic immunotherapies, to obtain an elevated level of immune activation. Following RFA, immunological responses are activated, and T-cells infiltrate the tumor. In patients with advanced HCC receiving tremelimumab, partial tumor ablation with RFA or TACE achieved a 26% and 89% response rate and disease control rate, respectively. Furthermore, 45% of stabilizations last longer than 26.07 weeks and have an OS of 53.45 weeks [22]. As a result of these encouraging findings, clinical trials involving the use of ICIs, whether alone or combined with other ICIs or bevacizumab, in accordance with chemo, radioembolization, or post-complete percutaneous or surgical ablation, have given considerable support.

6. Reactions and resistivity

It is critical to developing pretreatment baseline levels of T-cell infiltration and stimulation when evaluating response to checkpoint inhibition in different carcinomas. While the influence of CD4+ and CD8 + T-cell infiltration on survival post advanced HCC treatment using second-line PD1 inhibitors has been observed in the form of poor interactions and trends. The underlined results show that the impact is not as significant as originally assumed. According to the immunohistochemistry results, about 20% of advanced HCC tumors express PDL1. Tumor responses were reported in the CheckMate 040 trial independent of PDL1 expression. However, response rates were higher in patients with a minimum of 1% of tumor cells expressing PDL1. PDL1 expression in stromal immune cells as well as in tumor cells was elevated in pembrolizumab-treated patients who obtained objective remission. However, according to the obtained results, the responses were observed even in the absence of expression in both types of cells. In naive patients associated with PDL1-positive HCC, median OS was 70 weeks and 37.3 weeks (HR 0.80), accordingly. In the case of PDL1-negative HCC patients, after sorafenib and nivolumab treatment, the median OS was 72.6 weeks and 66 weeks (HR 0.84), respectively. Furthermore, a trend toward better OS with nivolumab monotherapy was observed in patients with increased tumor infiltration via CD3 + or CD8 + cells. In addition, various signatures of inflammatory genes (such as COX-2) were linked to an elevated response rate and OS. The underlined gene signatures were linked to inflammatory activities, cytolytic genes, IFN-associated genes, exhaustion markers, NK cell markers, and antigen presentation. In this view, these findings reveal an elevated level and activity of T cells and NK cells that utilize cytolysis and IFNγ as their primary antitumor effector mechanisms. In this study, the most complicated transcriptome classification, which includes a huge set of genes, was not found to be predictive of response. However, in the current evaluation, the number of patients for whom small data of RNA sequencing were existing, as large sample data could provide more definitive outcomes (positive or negative). Integrating genomics and transcriptomics into immunotherapy effectiveness will include comprehensive integrative analysis as well as obtaining biopsy samples before and during therapy.

Patients with objective remissions demonstrated potent CD3 + and CD8 + infiltration as compared with non-responders in paired HCC biopsy samples taken prior to and post two doses of tremelimumab. In the case of the combinations, objective HCC remissions were achieved regardless of PDL1 expression in nivolumab + ipilimumab treated cancerous cells. A single biomarker is insufficiently sensitive to provide timely clinical data. However, thorough immunohistological, mutational, and transcriptomic evaluations are required, as integrated multifactorial indices may be able to determine subgroups of individuals who would take advantage of ICI treatment. The significance of matching biopsies prior to and following treatment cannot be emphasized, since diagnostic biopsies for HCC are rarely taken.

The question of whether we are dealing with synergistic effects or just an additive impact arises when evaluating the enhanced combination of ICI therapeutic efficacy. Complementary analysis from major clinical studies is still lacking. Nevertheless, a subgroup analysis has reported a correlation between durvalumab, tremelimumab, or both in combinations. Furthermore, on day 15 after therapy began, an elevated level of proliferating Ki67 + CD8 + T cells among blood mononuclear cells was observed. In particular, in comparison with durvalumab, tremelimumab monotherapies, or the combined effect of a routine low dosage of tremelimumab with a similar dosage of durvalumab, the elevation in the underlined population of peripheral effector T-cells was found optimum for responders to an elevated priming dosage of durvalumab plus tremelimumab. The underlined combined therapies obtained the highest OS. It could be helpful to use biomarkers that are easily available to help design new combinations of therapies and to compare data between combinations. Significant TME changes were found in animal models with VEGFR blockade. The blockage of VEGFR improves PD1 inhibitory activity. According to multiple reported studies on mouse models, combined VEGFR and PD1 inhibition decreases M2-polarized macrophages and T-reg cells, enhances HCC cells and PDL1 expression in TAMs, and enhances normalized vasculature development triggered by CD4 + cells. Notably, effectiveness was achieved with a low dosage of anti-angiogenics (vascular normalizing rather than anti-vascular), offering a promising path of research into minimizing the associated toxicities.

The development of ADAs (anti-drug antibodies) that can affect the elimination of these drugs or neutralize their effectiveness is another viable cause of tumor resistance. The estimated prevalence of ADAs during monotherapies with anti-CTLA4 (ipilimumab), anti-PD1 (cemiplimab, nivolumab, and pembrolizumab), and anti-PDL1 (durvalumab and avelumab) agents is low, ranging from 0 to 12.7% in all tumor types. While no relevant impact of ADAs on efficiency has been noticed for nivoluma. ADAs, on the other hand, were found in up to 36% of NSCLC patients who had received atezolizumab and had a negative impact on systemic exposure to the drug as well as antitumor effectiveness. In the case of HCC, effectiveness (impact on OS) was poorer in the 20% of patients (ADA-positive by week 6) treated with bevacizumab and atezolizumab in a subanalysis of the IMbrave150 study. PD-L1 and CTLA4 are only two molecules that are involved in T cell exhaustion. There are many others on the surface of tumor cells that could compensate. Also, CTLs may have a hard time penetrating solid tumors, especially those that are encased in a fibrous capsule. This may also limit the effects of immunotherapy.

7. Management of immunotherapy toxicities

7.1 Immune-associated side effects

Immune checkpoints or coinhibitory receptors including CTLA-4 and PD-1 control T cell reactions and are efficient therapeutic targets [37, 38]. One of the drawbacks of the underlined advancements in the development of a novel spectrum of immune-related adverse events (irAEs), which are frequently distinct from the conventional toxicities associated with chemotherapy. Due to the rising use of ICIs in oncology, clinicians will progressively encounter both frequent and rare irAEs; hence, it is needed to increase attention regarding the clinical manifestation, evaluation, and managing these toxicities.

Unlike anti-CTLA-4-related adverse events, the risk of irAEs caused by PD-1/PD-L1 inhibition is independent of dosage [39, 40]. The skin and gastrointestinal tract were the most commonly affected organ systems by anti-CTLA4 and PD-1/PD-L1 inhibitors, whereas the liver and the endocrine system were less frequently damaged [39, 40]. However, ipilimumab was found to be linked with a considerably elevated incidence of rash and colitis than anti-PD-1/PD-L1 medicines [41].

7.2 irAEs management

Since irAEs are linked with a large array of aggravating conditions in the HCC, hepatologists face numerous hurdles while detecting and treating them. First, liver cirrhosis causes immunological dysfunction, which worsens over time [42]. Consequently, the immunological homeostasis linked with the liver in these patients is substantially damaged. Second, cirrhosis-related hepatic and extrahepatic consequences may overlap with or intensify symptoms mediated by irAEs [43]. Consequently, prior to ICI therapy, HCC patients should be carefully selected and evaluated [43].

Furthermore, the underlined approaches should be utilized for managing irAEs. First, strict surveillance is required, with weekly clinical controls, based on the intensity of the incidents. This is especially critical in patients with liver cirrhosis because distinguishing between problems (linked with cirrhosis) and irAEs can be difficult, and prematurely terminating a considerable antitumor therapy or initiating steroid therapy in cirrhotic patients might have serious implications [43].

Depending on the nature and severity of irAEs, it may be required to temporarily stop or permanently discontinue ICI therapy. With the exception of PD-1/PD-L1-driven rash, nephritis, adrenal insufficiency, and hypothyroidism, which recover after 1 month of treatment, permanent termination of ICI therapy should be addressed for irAEs of grade ≥ 3 [43]. There is a considerable risk of recurrence of irAEs when ICI medication is restarted after it has been discontinued: Twenty-five percent (22 of 40) of the 93 patients with irAEs of grade ≥ 2 who were treated with anti-PD-1/PD-L1 drugs had a recurrence of irAEs post-termination [44]. While recurrence of irAEs was linked with a more rapid onset of the early irAE, the frequency of the recurring irAEs did not vary [44]. TKIs used for HCC include sorafenib, lenvatinib, regorafenib and cabozantinib, all of which are associated with skin toxicity. However, the type of adverse effect and time course can help distinguish between ICI- and TKI-related events. For TKIs, the onset of rash is usually within weeks of starting and palmar-plantar erythema is the most common AE, reported in 52% and 27% of patients receiving sorafenib and lenvatinib, respectively. 29 This compares with around 2% for PD1 inhibitors. Additionally, the relatively short half-life of TKIs results in rapid resolution of skin toxicity over the course of days, which contrasts with the weeks or months that may be required for ICI-related toxicity to resolve.

Glucocorticoids may be prescribed for irAEs of grade ≥ 2 (0.5–2 mg/kg/day prednisone PO or IV, depending on the kind and intensity of the irAEs). Topical, oral, and intravenous glucocorticoids, as well as oral or topical antihistamines, are used to treat cutaneous irAEs, which range from simple rash or itch to less common but more serious illnesses such as Stevens-Johnson syndrome (SJS) [43]. Stevens-Johnson syndrome (SJS) is a form of severe adverse drug reactions and is characterized by epidermal necrolysis. The disease has the unique expression of blisters on the skin and the affection of mucous membranes in the mouth, nose, eyes, and genitals. SJS is characterized by a large area of skin and mucosal epithelial cell shedding and typical performance on the oropharynx, eyes, urogenitals, and anal mucosa. SJS has less than 10% of body surface area involvement. Steroids should be continued for at least 3 days before being reduced over 1–4 weeks [21, 45]. It should be noted that steroids are only beneficial in non-viral-associated chronic liver disease. If viruses are involved (HBV, HCV), steroids will simply permit virus replication to increase, and when steroids are withdrawn, a severe exacerbation of chronic liver disease may be seen.

Differential diagnosis is required for gastrointestinal irAEs, notably colitis and/or diarrhea, to rule out infectious illnesses and medication adverse effects [43]. For grades 2 and ≥ 3, glucocorticoids should be started, and hospitalization with sigmoidoscopy/colonoscopy should be considered. Moreover, immunosuppressive medication should be added early in the case of glucocorticoid failure [43, 46]. Depending on the steroid reaction and the severity of clinical presentation, discontinuation should be done over 2–8 weeks [21, 45].

Immune-related hepatitis is particularly difficult to diagnose and treat in individuals with HCC who are receiving ICI therapy [43]. However, early contact with an experienced hepatologist is thus strongly advised. Intrahepatic growth of the tumor, HBV/HCV flares, and adverse events linked with hepatotoxic medication, ascites, cholestasis, and CMV reactivation should all be ruled out before a diagnosis of immune-associated hepatitis is made. A liver biopsy should also be conducted prior to the administration of steroids [43].

Pneumonitis is an irAE that can be life-threatening. Hence, a prompt and extensive differential diagnosis should be conducted with suspected pneumonitis, including the exclusion of portopulmonary hypertension, viral etiologies, and hepatopulmonary syndrome [43]. Steroids should be started for grade 2 and discontinued over a period of 4–6 weeks [21]. Post glucocorticoid failure, infliximab (which is inflammatory by inhibiting TNFα) or mycophenolate mofetil (an immunosuppressive compound that inhibits inosine monophosphate dehydrogenase) may be administered [43]. It should be noted that therapeutic approaches involving prolonged immunosuppression increase the risk for selected infectious diseases and tumor types that usually never develop in the presence of intact immune surveillance.

8. Future directions

The licensing of the initial ICIs in advanced HCC and their clinical efficacy have revolutionized the concept of cancer immunotherapy. However, this field still has to address three major questions: Is immunotherapy beneficial in the preclinical stage? If so, it will reduce the risk of disease progression to cancer. In addition to PD-1/PD-L1/CTLA-4 suppression, which immunological treatments have antitumor effects in HCC? Which therapy options exist for patients not responding to the presently approved ICIs? Perhaps immunomodulation with histone deacetylase inhibitors (HDACi) in combination with ICI would permit a sustained antitumor response with reduced risk of adverse effects.

In response to the first question, various clinical studies in the initial and intermediate stages have reported the use of ICIs. It's uncertain whether checkpoint inhibitor exhibit regimens are a TACE alternative. As an alternative, the RENOTACE and ABC-HCC trials will test atezolizumab with bevacizumab and regorafenib plus nivolumab. Patients above the up-to-seven criteria, i.e., the subgroup with a relatively great tumor burden at an advanced stage, were recruited for RENOTACE, whereas patients with the whole spectrum of intermediate stages of disease were targeted for ABC-HCC. In addition, the initial trials examining ICIs for neoadjuvant approaches are currently in progress. The underlined collection of trials will look at the safety and efficacy of immunotherapy in the initial and intermediate stages from a variety of perspectives, providing high-quality data that will be useful in understanding the contribution of ICIs in the underlined situations.

To address the second question, there are a number of treatments that are currently being evaluated in clinical trials, which include the use of oncolytic viruses, CAR T/NK cells, and LAG-3 checkpoint inhibitors. These treatments might help patients with established ICIs who are unresponsive or have failed to respond to the treatment.

The third question may also be addressed by the above new immunotherapeutic strategies. A subset of patients, particularly those with an immunological desert TME, is likely to take advantage less of immunotherapy. Although immunotherapy has made tremendous advances. It should not be overlooked when considering treatment options for patients who may benefit from existing and future specialized therapies.

Acknowledgements

This manuscript is supported by Natural Science Foundation of Shandong Province (ZR2021MH022).

Competing interests

No competing interests exist among the authors.

Keypoints

Based on the outcomes of recent clinical trials, it appears that a single agent may not be sufficient for treating HCC; consequently, combination therapy characterizes an important area of research for the systemic treatment of advanced HCC. Moreover, ICIs are now being considered as part of HCC treatments, and their use in combination with molecular targeted therapy is shown to be an effective way to boost the immune system's response. The combined therapy of atezolizumab/bevacizumab is the first-line treatment to receive regulatory approval.

Immune checkpoint inhibitors (ICIs) may potentially be effective at earlier stages of illness. Combination therapies are being investigated in the intermediate stage in combination with or in place of transarterial chemotherapy, which is currently the standard of care. ICIs are also being explored as adjuvant and neoadjuvant therapy in the setting of early and very early surgery or ablation.

New research reveals that the control of the commensal gut microbiome and hepatic antitumor immunity are linked. Moreover, ICIs have been linked to immune-related side effects. In HCC clinical studies, however, the prevalence of grade 3/4 incidents was moderate. Therefore, ICIs are largely considered to be a choice in advanced HCC patients.

Author details

Shihai Liu
Medical Research Center, The Affiliated Hospital of Qingdao University, Qingdao, Shandong, P.R. China

*Address all correspondence to: shliumed@126.com

References

[1] European Association for the Study of the Liver. Electronic address eee, European Association for the Study of the L: EASL clinical practice guidelines: Management of hepatocellular carcinoma. Journal of Hepatology. 2018;**69**:182-236

[2] Nault JC, Sutter O, Nahon P, et al. Percutaneous treatment of hepatocellular carcinoma: State of the art and innovations. Journal of Hepatology. 2018;**68**:783-797

[3] Llovet JM, Real MI, Montana X, et al. Arterial embolisation or chemoembolisation versus symptomatic treatment in patients with unresectable hepatocellular carcinoma: A randomised controlled trial. Lancet. 2002;**359**:1734-1739

[4] Binnewies M, Roberts EW, Kersten K, et al. Understanding the tumor immune microenvironment (TIME) for effective therapy. Nature Medicine. 2018;**24**:541-550

[5] Gajewski TF, Schreiber H, Fu YX. Innate and adaptive immune cells in the tumor microenvironment. Nature Immunology. 2013;**14**:1014-1022

[6] Topalian SL, Drake CG, Pardoll DM. Immune checkpoint blockade: A common denominator approach to cancer therapy. Cancer Cell. 2015;**27**:450-461

[7] Waldman AD, Fritz JM, Lenardo MJ. A guide to cancer immunotherapy: From T cell basic science to clinical practice. Nature Reviews. Immunology. 2020;**20**:651-668

[8] Finn RS, Qin S, Ikeda M, et al. Atezolizumab plus bevacizumab in unresectable hepatocellular carcinoma. The New England Journal of Medicine. 2020;**382**:1894-1905

[9] Llovet JM, Kelley RK, Villanueva A, et al. Hepatocellular carcinoma. Nature Review Diseases Primers. 2021;**7**:6

[10] Roayaie S, Obeidat K, Sposito C, et al. Resection of hepatocellular cancer </=2 cm: Results from two Western centers. Hepatology. 2013;**57**:1426-1435

[11] Hoechst B, Ormandy LA, Ballmaier M, et al. A new population of myeloid-derived suppressor cells in hepatocellular carcinoma patients induces CD4(+)CD25(+)Foxp3(+) T cells. Gastroenterology. 2008;**135**:234-243

[12] Arihara F, Mizukoshi E, Kitahara M, et al. Increase in CD14+HLA-DR −/low myeloid-derived suppressor cells in hepatocellular carcinoma patients and its impact on prognosis. Cancer Immunology, Immunotherapy. 2013;**62**:1421-1430

[13] Gao Q, Wang XY, Qiu SJ, et al. Overexpression of PD-L1 significantly associates with tumor aggressiveness and postoperative recurrence in human hepatocellular carcinoma. Clinical Cancer Research. 2009;**15**:971-979

[14] Xiao YS, Gao Q, Xu XN, et al. Combination of intratumoral invariant natural killer T cells and interferon-gamma is associated with prognosis of hepatocellular carcinoma after curative resection. PLoS One. 2013;**8**:e70345

[15] Anitei MG, Zeitoun G, Mlecnik B, et al. Prognostic and predictive values of the immunoscore in patients with rectal cancer. Clinical Cancer Research. 2014;**20**:1891-1899

[16] Gabrielson A, Wu Y, Wang H, et al. Intratumoral CD3 and CD8 T-cell densities associated with relapse-free survival in HCC. Cancer Immunology Research. 2016;**4**:419-430

[17] Bruix J, Takayama T, Mazzaferro V, et al. Adjuvant sorafenib for hepatocellular carcinoma after resection or ablation (STORM): A phase 3, randomised, double-blind, placebo-controlled trial. The Lancet Oncology. 2015;**16**:1344-1354

[18] Topalian SL, Taube JM, Pardoll DM. Neoadjuvant checkpoint blockade for cancer immunotherapy. Science. 2020;**2020**:367

[19] Liu J, Blake SJ, Yong MC, et al. Improved efficacy of neoadjuvant compared to adjuvant immunotherapy to eradicate metastatic disease. Cancer Discovery. 2016;**6**:1382-1399

[20] Gassmann D, Weiler S, Mertens JC, et al. Liver allograft failure after nivolumab treatment-a case report with systematic literature research. Transplantation Direct. 2018;**4**:e376

[21] Brahmer JR, Lacchetti C, Schneider BJ, et al. Management of Immune-Related Adverse Events in patients treated with immune checkpoint inhibitor therapy: American Society of Clinical Oncology clinical practice guideline. Journal of Clinical Oncology. 2018;**36**:1714-1768

[22] Liao Y, Wang B, Huang ZL, et al. Increased circulating Th17 cells after transarterial chemoembolization correlate with improved survival in stage III hepatocellular carcinoma: A prospective study. PLoS One. 2013;**8**:e60444

[23] Pinato DJ, Murray SM. Trans-arterial chemoembolization as a loco-regional inducer of immunogenic cell death in hepatocellular carcinoma: Implications for immunotherapy. Journal for Immunotherapy of Cancer. 2021;**9**: e003311

[24] Pinato DJ, Karamanakos G, Arizumi T, et al. Dynamic changes of the inflammation-based index predict mortality following chemoembolisation for hepatocellular carcinoma: A prospective study. Alimentary Pharmacology & Therapeutics. 2014;**40**:1270-1281

[25] Duffy AG, Ulahannan SV, Makorova-Rusher O, et al. Tremelimumab in combination with ablation in patients with advanced hepatocellular carcinoma. Journal of Hepatology. 2017;**66**:545-551

[26] Hack SP, Spahn J, Chen M, et al. IMbrave 050: A phase III trial of atezolizumab plus bevacizumab in high-risk hepatocellular carcinoma after curative resection or ablation. Future Oncology. 2020;**16**:975-989

[27] El-Khoueiry AB, Sangro B, Yau T, et al. Nivolumab in patients with advanced hepatocellular carcinoma (CheckMate 040): An open-label, non-comparative, phase 1/2 dose escalation and expansion trial. Lancet. 2017;**389**:2492-2502

[28] Kelley RK, Sangro B, Harris W, et al. Safety, efficacy, and pharmacodynamics of Tremelimumab plus Durvalumab for patients with unresectable hepatocellular carcinoma: Randomized expansion of a phase I/II study. Journal of Clinical Oncology. 2021;**39**:2991-3001

[29] Hegde PS, Wallin JJ, Mancao C. Predictive markers of anti-VEGF and emerging role of angiogenesis inhibitors as immunotherapeutics. Seminars in Cancer Biology. 2018;**52**:117-124

[30] Ren Z, Xu J, Bai Y, et al. Sintilimab plus a bevacizumab biosimilar (IBI305)

versus sorafenib in unresectable hepatocellular carcinoma (ORIENT-32): A randomised, open-label, phase 2-3 study. The Lancet Oncology. 2021;**22**:977-990

[31] Yau T, Kang YK, Kim TY, et al. Efficacy and safety of nivolumab plus ipilimumab in patients with advanced hepatocellular carcinoma previously treated with sorafenib: The CheckMate 040 randomized clinical trial. JAMA Oncology. 2020;**6**:e204564

[32] Finn RS, Ikeda M, Zhu AX, et al. Phase Ib study of Lenvatinib plus pembrolizumab in patients with unresectable hepatocellular carcinoma. Journal of Clinical Oncology. 2020;**38**:2960-2970

[33] Xu J, Zhang Y, Jia R, et al. Anti-PD-1 antibody SHR-1210 combined with Apatinib for advanced hepatocellular carcinoma, gastric, or esophagogastric junction Cancer: An open-label, dose escalation and expansion study. Clinical Cancer Research. 2019;**25**:515-523

[34] Butterfield LH, Ribas A, Dissette VB, et al. A phase I/II trial testing immunization of hepatocellular carcinoma patients with dendritic cells pulsed with four alpha-fetoprotein peptides. Clinical Cancer Research. 2006;**12**:2817-2825

[35] Moehler M, Heo J, Lee HC, et al. Vaccinia-based oncolytic immunotherapy Pexastimogene Devacirepvec in patients with advanced hepatocellular carcinoma after sorafenib failure: A randomized multicenter phase IIb trial (TRAVERSE). Oncoimmunology. 2019;**8**:1615817

[36] Magnolo N, Kingo K, Laquer V, et al. A phase 3 open-label, randomized multicenter study to evaluate efficacy and safety of secukinumab in pediatric patients with moderate to severe plaque psoriasis: 24-week results. Journal of the American Academy of Dermatology. 2022;**86**:122-130

[37] Keir ME, Butte MJ, Freeman GJ, et al. PD-1 and its ligands in tolerance and immunity. Annual Review of Immunology. 2008;**26**:677-704

[38] Rowshanravan B, Halliday N, Sansom DM. CTLA-4: A moving target in immunotherapy. Blood. 2018;**131**:58-67

[39] Wang PF, Chen Y, Song SY, et al. Immune-related adverse events associated with anti-PD-1/PD-L1 treatment for malignancies: A Meta-analysis. Frontiers in Pharmacology. 2017;**8**:730

[40] Bertrand A, Kostine M, Barnetche T, et al. Immune related adverse events associated with anti-CTLA-4 antibodies: Systematic review and meta-analysis. BMC Medicine. 2015;**13**:211

[41] De Velasco G, Je Y, Bosse D, et al. Comprehensive Meta-analysis of key immune-related adverse events from CTLA-4 and PD-1/PD-L1 inhibitors in Cancer patients. Cancer Immunology Research. 2017;**5**:312-318

[42] Albillos A, Lario M, Alvarez-Mon M. Cirrhosis-associated immune dysfunction: Distinctive features and clinical relevance. Journal of Hepatology. 2014;**61**:1385-1396

[43] Sangro B, Chan SL, Meyer T, et al. Diagnosis and management of toxicities of immune checkpoint inhibitors in hepatocellular carcinoma. Journal of Hepatology. 2020;**72**:320-341

[44] Simonaggio A, Michot JM, Voisin AL, et al. Evaluation of Readministration of immune checkpoint inhibitors after immune-related adverse events in patients with Cancer. JAMA Oncology. 2019;**5**:1310-1317

[45] Haanen J, Carbonnel F, Robert C, et al. Management of toxicities from immunotherapy: ESMO Clinical Practice Guidelines for diagnosis, treatment and follow-up. Annals of Oncology. 2017;**28**:iv119-iv142

[46] Abu-Sbeih H, Ali FS, Wang X, et al. Early introduction of selective immunosuppressive therapy associated with favorable clinical outcomes in patients with immune checkpoint inhibitor-induced colitis. Journal for Immunotherapy of Cancer. 2019;**7**:93

Chapter 7

Mechanisms of Hepatocarcinogenesis Development in an Acidic Microenvironment

Cheng Jin, You-Yi Liu and Bo-Shi Wang

Abstract

Liver cancer represents one of the most common solid tumors globally. Despite curative improvements made in liver cancer therapy these years, the 5-year survival rate of liver cancer remains poor. Understanding the mechanisms involved in the initiation and progression of liver cancer is essential for optimizing therapeutic strategies. In recent years, it has been discovered that the acidic tumor microenvironment attributed to increased glycolysis, and hypoxia contributes to liver cancer progression through promoting cancer cell proliferation, metabolic adaptation, and migration and invasion. In this paper, research advances in the mechanisms of hepatocarcinogenesis development under an acidic microenvironment are reviewed.

Keywords: liver cancer, hepatocarcinogenesis, mechanism, acidic tumor microenvironment

1. Introduction

Liver cancer is the sixth most frequently identified cancer and the third most common cause of cancer death worldwide [1]. As the early diagnosis of liver cancer is difficult, most patients are diagnosed at advanced stages and even accompanied with tumor metastasis. It is critical to fully understand the molecular mechanisms of liver cancer metastasis, which would be helpful to improve the early diagnosis, treatment, and prognosis of liver cancer patients [2]. It has been reported that abnormal blood perfusion and hypoxia, coupled with a glycolytic phenotype, generate acidic microenvironment, which promotes cancer cell proliferation, metabolic adaptation, and migration and invasion, playing an important role in tumor development and progression. However, the molecular mechanisms that coordinate the formation of the acidic microenvironment in liver cancer remain to be adequately studied [3]. Given that the tumor treatment strategies targeting acidic microenvironment contribute to the management of many tumors types [4], the study of key molecular elements affecting the acidic microenvironment is of great importance for the diagnosis and intervention of liver cancer. This paper reviews the relevant research mechanisms of hepatocarcinogenesis and development under the acidic microenvironment, aiming to provide novel insight for further research studies.

2. Development of the tumor acidic microenvironment

The acidic microenvironment is mainly produced by tumor energy metabolism and hypoxia in solid tumors. Stephen Paget proposed the "seed and soil" hypothesis, stating that metastasizing cancer cells "seed" only in certain especially hospitable tissues, akin to seeding in "fertile soil" [5]. Since then, subsequent studies have revealed several classes of metastasis causes, including the tumor acidic microenvironment. In the 1920s, Otto Warburg first described a phenomenon that cancer cells displayed an altered metabolism, attaining energy through glycolysis at disproportionately high rates even under hypoxic conditions (**Figure 1**) [6]. Glucose is converted into lactic acid through glycolysis. Nevertheless, energy can still be obtained through the glutaminolysis pathway instead of glycolysis. From both pathways, high amounts of lactic acid are generated and subsequently discharged into the extracellular space between cancer cells [7, 8]. Some key transporters and enzymes, including ras, src, p53, glut, etc., are regulated in cancer cells to ensure that the impact of expanded H^+ is removed. These changes enhance the rate of glucose uptake to support the rapid proliferation of tumor cells [4].

Hypoxia-inducible factors cannot be effectively degraded by enzymes under hypoxic conditions that are mainly caused by the rapid proliferation of tumor cells, resulting in stable and sustained expression in tumor cells [9]. The proliferation, invasion, migration, and energy metabolism of tumor cells are affected by these changes.

2.1 Energy metabolism

Normal cells consume oxygen for energy production. Liver cancer aerobic glycolysis, otherwise known as the Warburg effect, to produce energy [10]. The end products of aerobic glycolysis contribute to the establishment of the acidic microenvironment.

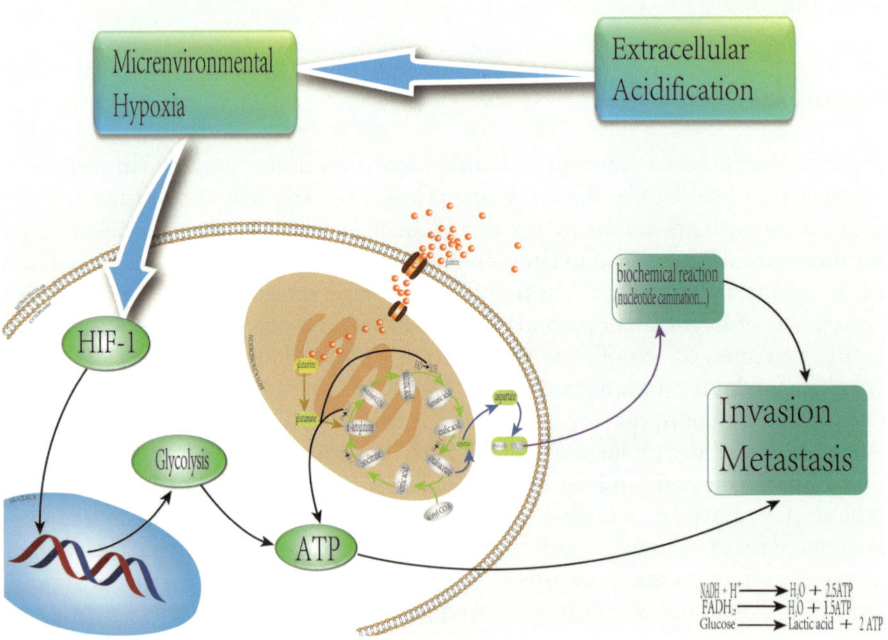

Figure 1.
Energy metabolism in acidic microenvironment.

In the acidic microenvironment, liver cancer cells regulate aerobic glycolysis by activating AMP-activated protein kinase (AMPK), PI3K/activity, and other related pathways, resulting in the increased expression of related proteins and enzymes, including glucose transporter, hexokinase, fructose-6-phosphate kinase, pyruvate kinase, and so on (**Figure 2**) [11]. As a carrier responsible for glucose transportation across the cell membrane, glucose transporter (GLUT) promotes higher glucose uptake in liver cancer cells [12]. Hexokinase, fructose-6-phosphate kinase, and pyruvate kinase are key enzymes of glycolysis. Relevant studies have shown that inhibition of the glucose transporter, hexokinase, and pyruvate kinase can attenuate the glucose metabolism of liver cancer cells, affecting the occurrence and development of liver cancer [13–16]. Upregulation of the activation ratio of phosphofructokinase [17] facilitates the adaptation of liver cancer cells to the microenvironment and accelerates the proliferation and growth of liver cancer cells. The energy needed for the proliferation of liver cancer cells is provided by these changes, and the same with the material basis required for establishment of the acidic microenvironment. By adopting a pattern of energy metabolism that is different from normal cells, the internal and external microenvironment of liver cancer cells is changed, improving their survival advantage. From this perspective, inhibiting the activity of glycolysis-related proteases in liver cancer cells may be an effective way to treat liver cancer.

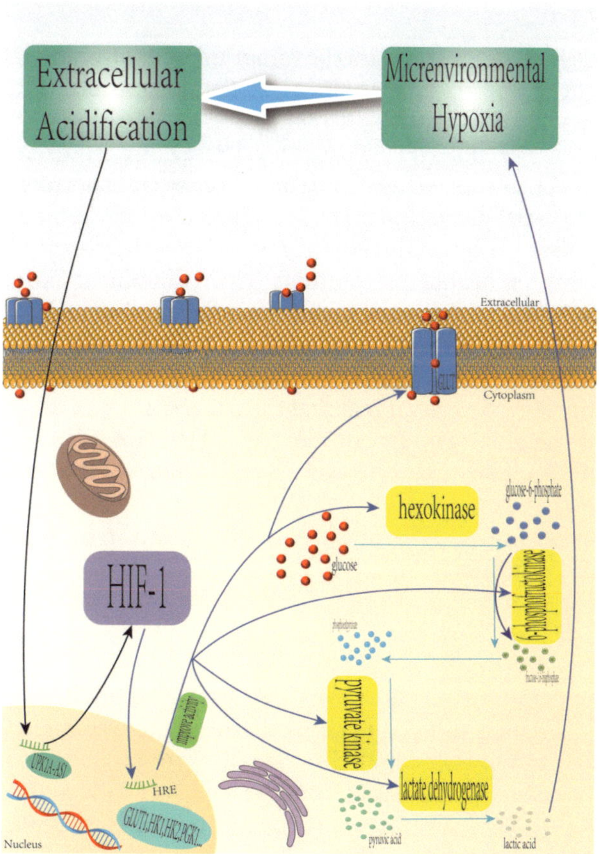

Figure 2.
Various enzymes related to glucose metabolism in acidic microenvironment.

2.2 Hypoxia

Hypoxia is a key feature of liver cancer, in which hypoxia-inducible factors (HIFs) play a key role [18, 19]. As the most studied hypoxia factor in liver cancer, the adaptive response of cells to the hypoxic microenvironment can be mediated by HIF-1, which is composed of HIF-1α and HIF-1β, as heterodimers that are expressed stably only in an anoxic environment but degraded rapidly in a normoxic environment [20, 21]. A variety of genes (such as Ras, C-MYC, p53, AMPK, etc.) and signaling pathways (such as PKB/Akt, PI3K, mTOR, etc.) can be transcriptionally regulated by HIF-1 and regulate the energy production of cancer cells to maintain their proliferation and survival [22]. It has been reported [23–26] that lactic acid production from of liver cancer cells can be amplified by HIF-1, which results in altering the activity of enzymes associated with glycolysis that lead to microenvironment acidification of liver cancer tissues. This inhibition can affect the growth and proliferation of liver cancer by regulating the energy metabolism. In addition, it has also been reported that liver cancer cells and tissues can upregulate the expression of HIF-1 and vascular endothelial growth factor (VEGF) during hypoxia [27–29]. VEGF is central for neovascularization of expanding tumor nodules.

3. Maintenance of tumor acidic microenvironment

The production of lactic acid causes the tumor microenvironment to be low in pH. Tumor cells excrete H^+ and acid metabolites into the extracellular environment to avoid intracellular acidosis (**Figure 3**). To achieve this goal, tumor cells use transporters that mainly include vacuolar-H^+ATPase (V-ATPase), Na^+/H^+ exchanger (NHE), monocarboxylic acid transporters (MCTs), bicarbonate transporters, and hydrochloric acid transporters to expel intracellular H^+. In addition, the carbonic anhydrases (CAs) can be used to regulate pH by catalyzing the reversible hydration of CO_2 to form bicarbonate and a proton in aqueous solutions. The reduction of extracellular pH is sensed by other complex mechanisms that include G-protein-coupled receptors, T-cell death-related gene 8 (TDAG8), acid-sensitive ion channels (ASICs), and the transient receptor potential channels, vanillin subfamily 1(TRPV1), to regulate the tumor microenvironment [30]. We can understand the occurrence and development of liver cancer and provide favorable conditions for targeted therapy of liver cancer by studying these transporters and complex pH-sensing molecular mechanisms in liver cancer.

3.1 Study on the mechanism of intracellular pH regulation of liver cancer in an acidic microenvironment

3.1.1 Vacuolar H^+-ATPase (V-ATPase)

Vacuolar H^+-adenosine triphosphatase (V-ATPase) is ubiquitously expressed in eukaryotic cells [31], being situated not only in the membranes of many organelles but also in the plasma membrane [32]. Studies have demonstrated that V-ATPase is functionally expressed in some human tumor cell lines and plays an important role in the regulation of tumor acidic microenvironment [33–35]. V-ATPase has multiple subunits, and the C subunit of V-ATPase, ATP6L, is the most thoroughly studied. Xu et al. [36] showed that the expression of ATP6L, the C subunit of V-ATPase, was elevated on the plasma membrane of liver cancer cells. As it indiscriminately inhibits

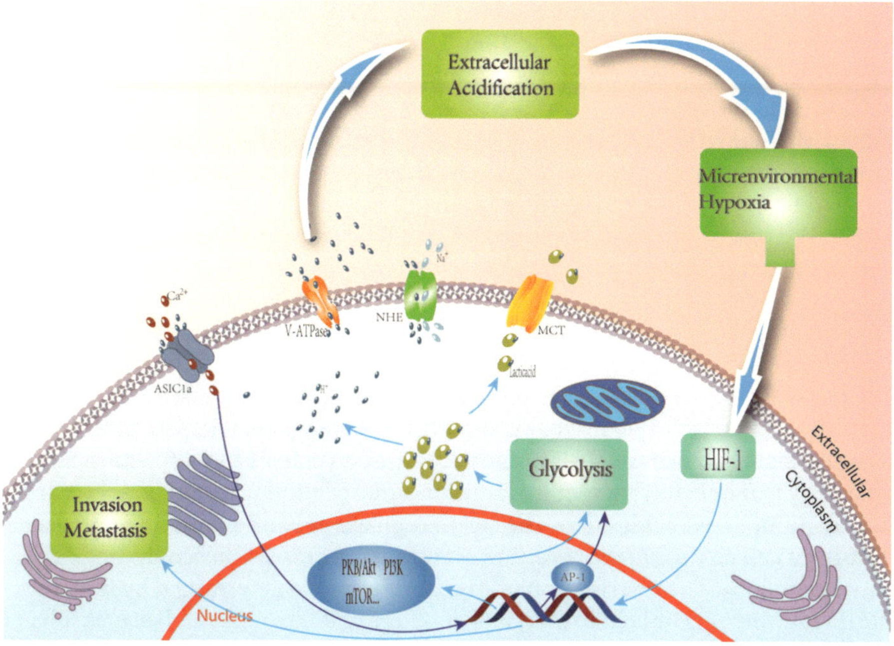

Figure 3.
Molecular mechanism of transport in acidic microenvironment.

V-ATPase in both mammals and non-mammals, palomycin was used to inhibit V-ATPase, thereby reducing the acid load and pH of liver cancer cells. Further, in an orthotopic xenograft model, the growth of liver cancer cells was delayed [37]. Tang et al. [38] showed that the protein expressed by LASS2 can bind to ATP6L and can inhibit the transmembrane transport of H^+ by V-ATPase proton pump. In this case, the mitochondrial apoptosis pathway is activated by increasing the concentration of hydrogen ions in the cell to induce apoptosis and inhibit the growth of tumor cells. These results imply that the expression of V-ATPase is increased in liver cancer cells and involved in the regulation of intracellular pH, while the growth of liver cancer cells can be effectively delayed by its corresponding inhibition.

3.1.2 Na^+/H^+ exchangers (NHEs)

Na^+/H^+ exchangers (NHEs) are a family of membrane proteins that contribute to exchanging one intracellular proton for one extracellular sodium. The family of NHEs consists of nine known members, NHE1-9. Each isoform represents a different gene product that has unique tissue expression, membrane localization, physiological effects, pathological regulation, and sensitivity to drug inhibitors [39]. NHE1 was the first to be discovered and is often referred to as the "housekeeping" isoform of the NHE family [40]. The NHE protein is activated by increased intracellular H^+, can achieve a one-to-one exchange between intracellular H^+ and extracellular Na^+, and excess Na^+ can be regulated by Na^+/K^+-ATPase in cells, which is a key ingredient in preventing cellular acidosis [40]. Enhanced glycolysis increases the amount of H^+ in cancer cells, by which the NHE protein is effectively activated. Yang et al. [41] showed that the expression of NHE1 was increased in liver cancer and in cells and closely related to tumor size, venous invasion, and tumor stage. Kim et al. [42] showed that curcumin combined with GR was used to inhibit NHE1 expression in liver cancer cells characterized by low pH. In addition, Li et al. [43] showed that the growth and metastasis of liver cancer cells can be inhibited by Ginsenoside (Rg3), which blocks the EGF-EGFR-ERK1/2-HIF pathway by decreasing the expression of NHE1. As these results imply that NHE1 is involved in regulating intracellular pH and is upregulated in liver cancer cells, inhibition of it can effectively delay tumor cell growth and metastasis. Further study of NHE1 may effectively inhibit the progression of liver cancer. However, the role of other subtypes of NHEs in liver cancer is unclear and needs to be further studied.

3.1.3 Monocarboxylic acid transporters (MCTs)

MCTs belong to the SLC16 gene family and consist of 14 members, in which MCT1, MCT2, and MCT4 can act as proton transporters to participate in the transport of pyruvate and lactate [44]. In the process of glycolysis a lot of lactic acid is produced by tumor cells that require large amounts of monocarboxylic acid transporters to pump these acids out of the cell to regulate pH and maintain homeostasis in the tumor cell environment, which prevents cell apoptosis caused by lactic acid accumulation [45]. The distribution of MCTs in tissues is determined by the physiological requirements of lactate metabolism (**Figure 4**). In general, because it has a high affinity for lactic acid, MCT1 and MCT4, which are expressed in most tissues, are mainly responsible for the transport of lactic acid inside cells. However, glucose metabolism determines the level of MCT2 expression, where its affinity for pyruvate is much higher than other MCTs molecules, and intracellular pyruvate transport is mainly completed by it. In some literature reports, MCT1 and MCT4 are highly expressed in liver cancer, and the high expression of it was significantly correlated with the malignant phenotype and prognosis of the tumor, but MCT2 expression is low in hepatocellular carcinoma [46, 47]. Chen et al. found that the expression of MCT4 was positively correlated with the expression of GLUT1 and speculated that

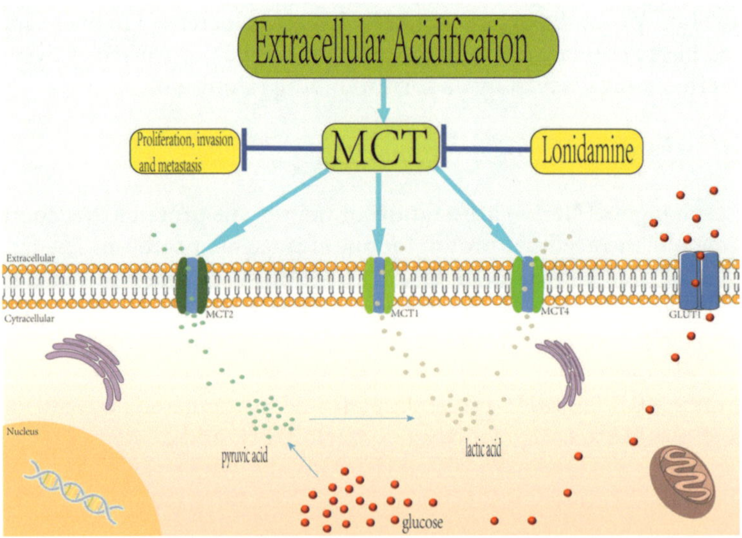

Figure 4.
Related mechanism of MCT in acidic microenvironment.

there was a positive feedback loop between the growth of HCC and the upregulation of MCT4/GLUT1 [48]. As an antitumor drug, lonidamine effectively inhibits MCTs, and it can impair the proliferation, metastasis, and invasion of liver cancer cells by reducing glycolysis [49]. These results imply that the specific molecular mechanism of MCTs involvement in the development of liver cancer may be related to MCTs mediating the shuttle of lactate and pyruvate in and out of liver cancer cells, which prevents lactic acid from accumulating in the liver cancer microenvironment and pyruvate from being transported extracellular that inhibits the proliferation and survival of HCC cells. However, the specific molecular pathways and related mechanisms remain unclear and need to be further studied.

3.1.4 Carbonic anhydrases (Cas)

Tumor tissues are often exposed to low oxygen that can activate CAs by which H_2O and CO_2 are reversibly converted to HCO_3 so that the chemical reaction can maintain the normal pH of the cell. CAs can be divided into four categories according to their distribution location (cell and subcellular) [50], namely cytoplasmic type (CAI, II, III, VII, XIII), mitochondrial type (cava, VB), secretory type (CAVI), and membrane-related type (CAIX, XII, XIV, XV). Among them, CAII and CAXII are the most studied in liver cancer. Xing et al. [51] showed that the expression of carbonic anhydrase II (CAII) was significantly upregulated in liver cancer compared with serum CAII concentrations in the normal population and among patients with non-recurrent liver cancer. Further investigating the molecular mechanisms involved suggests that CaII increases the migration and invasion of liver cancer cells by activating the epithelial-mesenchymal transition (EMT) pathway. Finkelmeier et al. [52] showed that the serum CAXII level was significantly increased in patients with advanced liver cancer (BCLC and ALBI scores). Zeng et al. [53] showed that the high expression of CAXII was associated with poor prognosis in patients with liver cancer. UDA et al. [54] showed that the changes in intracellular pH can be caused by knocking out CAII, which inhibits the progression of liver cancer. Han et al. [55] showed that the proliferation of liver cancer can be inhibited by tiliroside by blocking CAXII. These findings suggest that CAXII may also be a prognostic indicator of poor prognosis in patients with liver cancer. The molecular mechanisms of CAII and CAXII affecting the progression of liver cancer need to be further explored, and the specific roles of other subtypes of CAs in the progression of liver cancer need to be further determined. However, according to current studies, CAII and CAXII may be potential treatment targets sites for liver cancer.

3.2 Study on the mechanism of extracellular pH regulation of liver cancer in an acidic microenvironment

3.2.1 Acid sensing ion channels (ASICs)

Changes in extracellular pH can be sensed by acid-sensitive ion channels (ASICs). Six ASICs subunits are encoded by four genes have been cloned, which comprise ASIC1a, 1B, 2A, 2B, 3, and 4 [56]. A large number of crucial biological functions, such as inflammation, ischemia, and tissue acidification of tumors, are represented in ASICs. ASIC1a is of particular interest as one of its six subunits that play an important physiological and pathological role from mediating Ca^{2+}influx [57]. Our team has been working on ASIC1a for many years since it is involved in the proliferation, invasion, and metastasis of liver cancer. When liver cancer tissues were in a pH 6.5 microenvironment, the expression of ASIC1a in liver cancer tissues was significantly higher than that in adjacent non-tumor tissues in previous studies [3]. ASIC1a protects against phosphorylation and ubiquitination of β-catenin and promotes β-catenin nuclear aggregation to stimulate the proliferation of HCC cells. ASIC1a can promote invasion and migration of liver cancer as demonstrated by cell scratch and trans-well assay data [58]. Downstream differentially expressed genes of ASIC1a were mainly concentrated in the transcription factor AP-1 in the MAPK-related signaling pathways [59]. These findings suggest that intracellular Ca^{2+} concentrations and changes in downstream AP-1 expression can be increased by ASIC1a to affect the migration and invasion of liver cancer. Thus, ASIC1a is an effective target for the treatment of liver cancer, and a precise study of the relevant mechanisms may provide a new diagnostic method or target.

3.2.2 Transient receptor potential channels vanillin subfamily 1 (TRPV1)

TRPV1 channel, which is a cation channel with high selectivity for Ca^{2+}, is activated by excessive extracellular H^+ in the absence of other stimuli [60]. Miao et al. [61] demonstrated that the high expression of TRPV1 in liver cancer patients with disease-free survival rate was significantly better than low TRPV1 expression from the variable analysis. In in vivo and in vitro experiments with dimethylnitrosamine (DEN)-induced gene models, combined with bioinformatics analysis of mouse and human liver cancer samples, were used to further study the molecular mechanism and related role of TRPV1 in liver cancer. The results showed that the liver microenvironment can be altered and the development of liver cancer be promoted from knockout of TRPV1 [62]. Some published papers have proved showed that TRPV1 can be activated by cannabinoid and capsaicin that may lead to apoptosis of liver cancer cells, which indicates that TRPV1 perhaps can be used as a therapeutic site and prognostic molecule for liver cancer [63].

4. Tumor acidic microenvironment and the progress of liver cancer

The complex molecular mechanisms that generate an acidic microenvironment of liver cancer also affect autophagy [64] as well as the role of exosomes [65] in the occurrence and development of liver cancer. and Liver cancer cells also demonstrate immune escape, thereby developing the ability to migrate and metastasize [4].

4.1 The acidic tumor microenvironment promotes invasion and metastasis of liver cancer

Although the acidic tumor microenvironment has been shown to promote cancer metastasis, its potential regulatory mechanism remains unclear. In recent years, it has been confirmed that exosomes play an increasingly important role in promoting the invasion and metastasis of liver cancer in the acidic microenvironment [66, 67]. Exosomes are membrane vesicles that are 30–100 nm in size and are released by various cell types into the extracellular environment. Although initially considered as "garbage transporters" from parental cells, exosomes are now recognized as a new category of intercellular communicators. Cells constitutively sort envelope proteins and RNAs into exosomes, a process that can be stimulated by a variety of pathologic stimuli [68]. Tian et al.'s results showed that acidic microenvironment increased liver cancer cell–derived exosomal miR-21 and miR-10b levels, which could promote migration and invasion of recipient liver cancer cells cultured under normal conditions both in vivo and in vitro [69]. It has also been reported that exosomes can promote the progression and metastasis of liver cancer through epithelial-mesenchymal transition (EMT), which is a process in which cells gradually lose the morphological characteristics of epithelial cells and transform into mesenchymal types, which is often related to tumor invasion and metastasis [70]. Xia et al. proved that the expression of receptor tyrosine kinase-like orphan receptor 1 was upregulated in the acidic microenvironment, which led to the metastasis and invasion of liver cancer by promoting EMT [71]. It is proposed that the acidic microenvironment can promote the invasion and metastasis of liver cancer through exosomes. On the other hand, Takahashi et al. confirm that exosomes can regulate HIF-1 by transporting lincror-α expression levels in response to hypoxic conditions [72]. Further, the acidification of the liver cancer microenvironment is increased by hypoxia, while angiogenesis is promoted in response to the stress created by hypoxia [73–75]. Jin et al. showed that hepatic stellate cells are activated by an acidic tumor microenvironment and subsequently promote liver cancer metastasis via osteopontin [76], which indicates that the invasion and metastasis of liver cancer are regulated by the acidic microenvironment. In general, exosomes may alter cell matrix and promote epithelial mesenchymal transformation of hepatocellular carcinoma cells through their role as intercellular transporters and enhance the invasion and metastasis of liver cancer by influencing the acidification of HIF-1 microenvironment. The invasion and metastasis of liver cancer are influenced by an acidic microenvironment, on which further study may find an effective method to inhibit metastasis and invasion of liver cancer.

4.2 Tumor acidic microenvironment and immune escape

Tumor immunity is emerging as a crucial factor in cancer control and treatment. Spontaneous immune responses arising in cancer patients have been proved to condition disease course and positively impact prognosis [77]. If tumor cells have intrinsic antigenicity, which means that they cannot avoid being recognized by specific immune cell subsets, they do learn quite quickly how to escape immune recognition. Developing sophisticated mechanisms to shut down immunological responses, cancer cells not only survive in an immune competent host, but they proliferate, progress locally and disseminate systemically, often overcoming the control attempts of immune defense [78]. In fact, innate and adaptive immune cells are highly sensitive to the hypoxic microenvironment characterized by most solid cancers. Studies have demonstrated that hypoxia induces the expression of a range of chemokines and cytokines, such as TGF-β, IL-8, CCL26, and so on, regulating the recruitment and polarization of macrophages and neutrophils and aggravating immunosuppression and evasion [79]. The increase of lactic acid caused by hypoxia can reduce T cell metabolism and affect T cell differentiation and function [80–85], by which NK cells can be inhibited and thus reduce NK cell production of IFN [86]. The tumor microenvironment can be further acidified by neutrophils by releasing an H^+-pump ATPase that block NK and T cell activity, neutrophil apoptosis of which can be delayed, the inflammatory response of neutrophils be maintained, and can also stimulate the release of TGF by tumor cells and some immune cells [87, 88]. It has also been reported that the immune checkpoint can be upregulated hypoxia in TME and tumor immune escape be promoted [89]. These studies suggest that immune escape from solid tumors may be influenced by the acidic microenvironment, thereby promoting tumor proliferation and metastasis. However, less research has been done on immune escape in the acidic microenvironment of liver cancer. The impact of immune escape on liver cancer in an acidic microenvironment may have great potential in the treatment of liver cancer.

4.3 Tumor acidic microenvironment and autophagy

Autophagy is a process wherein the double membrane is shed from the rough surface endoplasmic reticulum of the ribosomal area and forms an autophagosome, which can envelop part of the cytoplasm and cell organelle protein composition and merge with a lysosome to form an autolysosome, which eventually degrades the autophagosome contents [90]. The process produces the energy or material a cancer cell needs to survive. Many studies have shown that autophagy plays an important role in normal cell maintenance and in tumorigenesis, drug resistance, and other pathophysiological processes [91–93]. The increased autophagy in solid tumors is an adaptive behavior in response to the harsh microenvironment [94]. Fan et al. had demonstrated that activating autophagy in liver cancer cells could increase glucose consumption and lactate production; Conversely, inhibition of autophagy resulted in reduced glucose consumption and lactate production. Further studies demonstrated that adding up regulates MCT1 expression and activates Wnt/β-Catenin signaling that could enhance glucose uptake and lactate production, so as to promote the metastasis and invasion of liver cancer [95]. Lin et al. provided evidence that autophagy modulates the level of glycolysis through ubiquitin-mediated selective degradation of HK2 [96]. Wang et al. study demonstrated that acidic TME confers liver cancer cells anoikis resistance via downregulation of miR-3663-3p and finally drives liver cancer metastasis [97]. These results suggest that autophagy is closely related to the occurrence and development of liver cancer. The invasion and metastasis of liver cancer are regulated by this adaptation to the environment. Further study of the mechanism of autophagy in an acidic microenvironment may be an effective way to treat liver cancer.

5. Perspectives of liver cancer therapy from tumor acidic microenvironment

The treatment of liver cancer is usually based on surgical treatment, of which early liver cancer can usually be resected, but systemic treatment of advanced liver cancer usually requires sorafenib in addition to local ablation, transcatheter chemoembolization, or external irradiation [98]. Multi-target tyrosine kinase inhibitor (TKI) Sorafenib has shown anti-angiogenesis and anti-proliferation effects in patients with advanced liver cancer and can inhibit tumor cell proliferation by inhibiting raf-1, B-Raf, and kinase activities in Ras/Raf/MEK/ERK signaling pathways, thus being used as an adjunctive therapy for advanced liver cancer [99, 100]. However, only approximately 30% of patients can benefit from sorafenib, and this population usually acquires drug resistance within 6 months [101]. Sorafenib inhibits the proliferation of liver cancer by anti-angiogenesis mainly by inhibiting the synthesis of hypoxia-inducible factor 1 (HIF-1), leading to the decrease of VEGF expression and tumor angiogenesis in liver cancer [102, 103]. A study by Liang et al. reported that hypoxia induced by continued sorafenib treatment conferred sorafenib resistance in liver cancer via HIF-1 and NF-κB activation [104]. Liver cancer glycolysis is promoted by this reverse-activated HIF-1, which further exacerbates the acidification of the microenvironment. It has also been reported that the structure and charge of drugs can be altered by acidic TME, which reduces their uptake by tumor cells and affects the delivery and efficacy of anticancer drugs as well as chemotherapy and radiotherapy [105, 106]. Therefore, the occurrence of sorafenib drug resistance may be caused, on the one hand, by the continuous treatment of hypoxia, which changes the expression of HIF-1 and increases drug resistance; but on the other hand, the change of HIF-1 aggravates the acidification of microenvironment, changes the physical and chemical properties of sorafenib to a certain extent, reduces the lethality of liver cancer, and aggravates the drug resistance of liver cancer. It has also been reported that changes in the microenvironment lead to increased resistance of gastric cancer cells to 5-fluorouracil and carboplatin [107]. Therefore, changes in the microenvironment are very important for the occurrence and development of tumors and drug treatment. It has been reported that urease can inhibit the development of human breast cancer and lung cancer by inducing extracellular pH alkalization [108]. Since the activity of immune cells can be inhibited by the acidification of microenvironment, the occurrence and development of tumor can be slowed down by using buffer to neutralize tumor acidosis and then immunotherapy, which has been reported in the literature as an effective method [109]. In addition, it has been reported that the progression of liver cancer can be slowed by inhibiting the activities of glycolic-related enzymes such as glucose transporter, hexokinase, pyruvate kinase, and 6-phosphofructokinase [12, 14, 16, 17]. Inhibition of V-ATPase by pavlomycin slowed the growth of liver cancer cells [37]. The growth and metastasis of liver cancer cells can be slowed down by inhibiting NHE1 activity, which can be inhibited by curcumin and GR in combination [42]. Lonidamine inhibits the proliferation, metastasis, and invasion of liver cancer cells by effectively inhibiting MCTs and thereby reducing glycolysis [49]. CAXII was inhibited by Tilroside and slowed down the proliferation of liver cancer [50]. The molecular mechanisms involved in glycolysis can be inhibited by these drugs, which inhibit the development of liver cancer. Therefore, the invasion and metastasis of liver cancer can be inhibited by changing the acidic microenvironment of liver cancer cells. Further study of the molecular mechanism of the acidic tumor microenvironment is a promising research direction for the treatment of liver cancer.

6. Conclusion and future perspectives

Acidic microenvironment is a common phenomenon in solid tumors [8]. It has been proved that microenvironmental acidification is a key step in transforming solid tumors from noninvasive to invasive [110]. The enhancement of glycolysis of tumor cells leads to obvious acidification of the tissue microenvironment. As one of the indispensable members of solid tumors, liver cancer is no exception, and the pH value of its microenvironment is usually around 6.5 [3]. As shown in **Figure 3**, the expression of enzymes mediating glycolysis in liver cancer cells is altered by microenvironmental acidification, which increases the expression of related proteins and glycolysis. However, the proliferation of liver cancer cells leads to widespread hypoxia in which hypoxia factors cannot normally be degraded in liver cancer cells. Glycolysis is promoted by changes in glycolic-related proteins and hypoxia factors by which vascular endothelial growth factor can be also promoted to stimulate the formation of blood vessels and the supply of glucose to liver cancer tissues and further promote glycolysis of liver cancer cells. Liver cancer cells activate intracellular related acid transporters to maintain the internal pH disturbance caused by intracellular acidification exacerbated by increased glycolysis. Extracellular H^+ excretion increases the extracellular hydrogen ion concentration, which activates extracellular hydrogen ion receptors such as ASICs, leading to further acidification of the liver cancer microenvironment. However, hydrogen ions cannot be discharged from cells indefinitely. When the regulation of hydrogen ions is impaired, TRPV1 will be actively activated in liver cancer tissue, by which cancer cells will be triggered into automatic apoptosis. On the other hand (**Figure 5**), epithelial-mesenchymal transition, invasion, and metastasis of hepatocellular carcinoma can be enhanced by selected exosomes that exchange information between hepatocellular carcinomas. Hypoxia-related factors can also further promote microenvironmental acidification. The activity of immune cells can be inhibited by an acidic microenvironment that causes the immune escape of liver cancer cells and facilitates the invasion and metastasis of liver cancer differently. The optimal pH value of the drug is changed by the acidification of the microenvironment that causes the tumors to develop drug resistance, which antitumor drugs generally have the right microenvironment to maximize their effects. Growth, proliferation, invasion, and metastasis of liver cancer are promoted by multiple molecular interactions implying that the liver cancer organization has accurate regulations and effective control and management.

However, the specific mechanism of the related molecules and their exact role in the development of liver cancer need to be understood in the acidic microenvironment (1) Whether there are differences in the activities of various molecular protein subtypes induced by the acidic microenvironment of liver cancer remains to be shown. Whether these proteins have been mutated in the acidic microenvironment of liver cancer cells, and if so, whether these mutations can promote the occurrence and development of liver cancer requires further investigation. (2) Related experiments

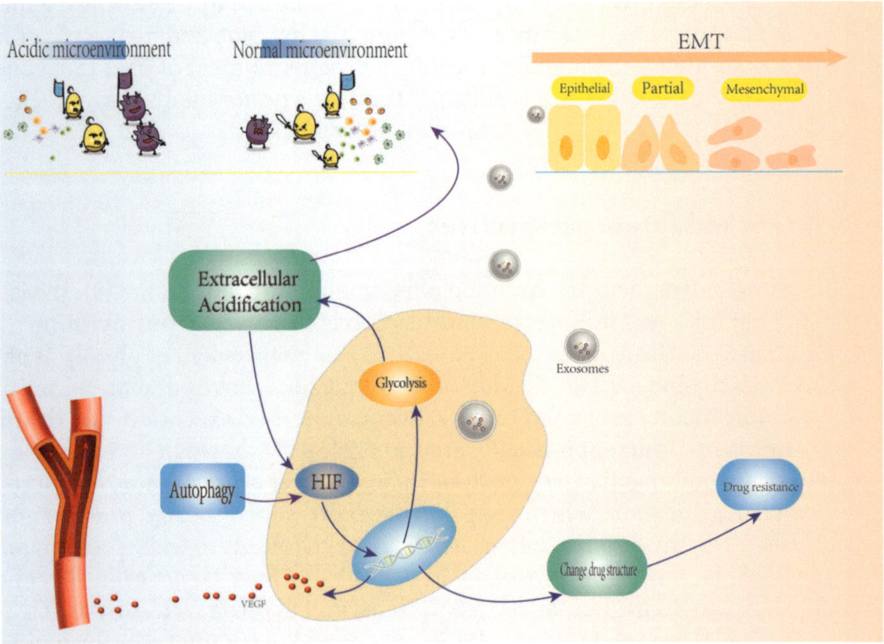

Figure 5.
Mechanism diagram of molecular changes in liver cancer tissue under acidic microenvironment.

have proved that drugs that inhibit the acidic microenvironment of hepatocellular carcinoma can inhibit the invasion and metastasis. Whether these drugs can be used clinically to inhibit metastasis and invasion of liver cancer will be the focus of future studies. (3) In the acidic microenvironment, the expression levels of these diagnostic molecules that include alpha-fetoprotein Lens Culinaris agglutin-3 (AFP-L3), alpha-fetoprotein (AFP), Des-γ-carboxy Prothrombin (DCP), and other molecules related to the diagnosis of liver cancer have not been reported [111]. In the acidic microenvironment of liver cancer, the activities of related enzymes that maintain pH were changed, which has been confirmed by many experiments. Can one or more of these enzymes be used as a diagnostic basis for early liver cancer?

Although surgical treatment of liver cancer is commonly practiced [112, 113], surgical treatment cannot fundamentally cure liver cancer, after which recurrence and metastasis rates remain high. This is a major reason why the molecular mechanism contributing to the occurrence and development of liver cancer is not well understood [114]. The mechanisms of liver cancer cell microenvironment acidification, and the identification of key genes that are differentially expressed under those conditions, may provide a new theoretical basis and molecular targets for the development of drugs that will treat liver cancer.

Acknowledgements

We are especially grateful for the training of 333 high-level talents in Jiangsu Province.

Conflict of interest

The authors declare no conflict of interests for this article.

Fund programs/support

333 High-level talents project of Jiangsu province (2022[2] in talent bureau of Jiangsu province); "Taihu lake" science and technology project of Wuxi (Y20212018); the first Outstanding Young and middle-aged Public Health talents project of Wuxi (BJ2020025).

Author details

Cheng Jin[1,2*], You-Yi Liu[2] and Bo-Shi Wang[1,2]

1 Department of Hepatobiliary Surgery, The Affiliated Hospital of Jiangnan University, Wuxi, Jiangsu Province, China

2 Wuxi School of Medicine in Jiangnan University, Wuxi, Jiangsu Province, China

*Address all correspondence to: jingcheng1008@163.com

References

[1] Liu Y, Zheng J, Hao J, et al. Global burden of primary liver cancer by five etiologies and global prediction by 2035 based on global burden of disease study 2019. Cancer Medicine. 2022;**11**:1310-1323. DOI: 10.1002/cam4.4551

[2] Han TS, Ban HS, Hur K, et al. The epigenetic regulation of HCC metastasis. International Journal of Molecular Sciences. 2018;**19**:3978. DOI: 10.3390/ijms19123978

[3] Jin C, Ye QH, Yuan FL, et al. Involvement of acid-sensing ion channel 1α in hepatic carcinoma cell migration and invasion. Tumour Biology. 2015;**36**:4309-4317. DOI: 10.1007/s13277-015-3070-6

[4] Boedtkjer E, Pedersen SF. The acidic tumor microenvironment as a driver of Cancer. Annual Review of Physiology. 2020;**82**:103-126. DOI: 10.1146/annurev-physiol-021119-034627

[5] Paget S. The distribution of secondary growths in cancer of the breast. 1889. Cancer Metastasis Reviews. 1989;**8**:98-101

[6] Warburg O, Wind F, Negelein E. The metabolism of tumors in the body. The Journal of General Physiology. 1927;**8**:519-530. DOI: 10.1085/jgp.8.6.519

[7] Zhang Y, Yang JM. Altered energy metabolism in cancer: A unique opportunity for therapeutic intervention. Cancer Biology & Therapy. 2013;**14**:81-89. DOI: 10.4161/cbt.22958

[8] Wang JX, Choi SYC, Niu X, et al. Lactic acid and an acidic tumor microenvironment suppress anticancer immunity. International Journal of Molecular Sciences. 2020;**21**:8363. DOI: 10.3390/ijms21218363

[9] Jing X, Yang F, Shao C, et al. Role of hypoxia in cancer therapy by regulating the tumor microenvironment. Molecular Cancer. 2019;**18**:157. DOI: 10.1186/s12943-019-1089-9

[10] Bustamante E, Pedersen PL. High aerobic glycolysis of rat hepatoma cells in culture: Role of mitochondrial hexokinase. Proceedings of the National Academy of Sciences of the United States of America. 1977;**74**:3735-3739. DOI: 10.1073/pnas.74.9.3735

[11] Feng J, Li J, Wu L, et al. Emerging roles and the regulation of aerobic glycolysis in hepatocellular carcinoma. Journal of Experimental & Clinical Cancer Research. 2020;**39**:126. DOI: 10.1186/s13046-020-01629-4

[12] Xiong T, Li Z, Huang X, et al. TO901317 inhibits the development of hepatocellular carcinoma by LXRα/Glut 1 decreasing glycometabolism. American Journal of Physiology. Gastrointestinal and Liver Physiology. 2019;**316**:G598-G607. DOI: 10.1152/ajpgi.00061.2018

[13] Chen X, She P, Wang C, et al. Hsa_circ_0001806 promotes glycolysis and cell progression in hepatocellular carcinoma through miR-125b/HK2. Journal of Clinical Laboratory Analysis. 2021;**35**:e23991. DOI: 10.1002/jcla.23991

[14] Yoo JJ, Yu SJ, Na J, et al. Hexokinase-II inhibition synergistically augments the anti-tumor efficacy of sorafenib in hepatocellular carcinoma. International Journal of Molecular Sciences. 2019;**20**:1292. DOI: 10.3390/ijms20061292

[15] Zhou Y, Lin F, Wan T, et al. ZEB1 enhances Warburg effect to facilitate

tumorigenesis and metastasis of HCC by transcriptionally activating PFKM. Theranostics. 2021;**11**:5926-5938. DOI: 10.7150/thno.56490

[16] Jia G, Wang Y, Lin C, et al. LNCAROD enhances hepatocellular carcinoma malignancy by activating glycolysis through induction of pyruvate kinase isoform PKM2. Journal of Experimental & Clinical Cancer Research. 2021;**40**:299. DOI: 10.1186/s13046-021-02090-7

[17] Golinska M, Troy H, Chung YL, et al. Adaptation to HIF-1 deficiency by upregulation of the AMP/ATP ratio and phosphofructokinase activation in hepatomas. BMC Cancer. 2011;**11**:198. DOI: 10.1186/1471-2407-11-198

[18] Yuen VW, Wong CC. Hypoxia-inducible factors and innate immunity in liver cancer. The Journal of Clinical Investigation. 2020;**130**:5052-5062. DOI: 10.1172/JCI137553

[19] Bao MH, Wong CC. Hypoxia, metabolic reprogramming, and drug resistance in liver Cancer. Cell. 2021;**10**:1715. DOI: 10.3390/cells10071715

[20] Liu Z, Wang Y, Dou C, et al. Hypoxia-induced up-regulation of VASP promotes invasiveness and metastasis of hepatocellular carcinoma. Theranostics. 2018;**8**:4649-4663. DOI: 10.7150/thno.26789

[21] Chu Q, Gu X, Zheng Q, Zhu H. Regulatory mechanism of HIF-1α and its role in liver diseases: A narrative review. Annals of Translational Medicine. 2022;**10**:109. DOI: 10.21037/atm-21-4222

[22] Moldogazieva NT, Mokhosoev IM, Terentiev AA. Metabolic heterogeneity of cancer cells: An interplay between HIF-1, GLUTs, and AMPK. Cancers (Basel). 2020;**12**:862. DOI: 10.3390/cancers12040862

[23] Savic LJ, Schobert IT, Peters D, et al. Molecular imaging of extracellular tumor pH to reveal effects of locoregional therapy on liver cancer microenvironment. Clinical Cancer Research. 2020;**26**:428-438. DOI: 10.1158/1078-0432.CCR-19-1702

[24] Maher JC, Wangpaichitr M, Savaraj N, et al. Hypoxia-inducible factor-1 confers resistance to the glycolytic inhibitor 2-deoxy-D-glucose. Molecular Cancer Therapeutics. 2007;**6**:732-741. DOI: 10.1158/1535-7163.MCT-06-0407

[25] Ma CN, Wo LL, Wang DF, et al. Hypoxia activated long non-coding RNA HABON regulates the growth and proliferation of hepatocarcinoma cells by binding to and antagonizing HIF-1 alpha. RNA Biology. 2021;**18**:1791-1806. DOI: 10.1080/15476286.2020.1871215

[26] Feng J, Dai W, Mao Y, et al. Simvastatin re-sensitizes hepatocellular carcinoma cells to sorafenib by inhibiting HIF-1α/PPAR-γ/PKM2-mediated glycolysis. Journal of Experimental & Clinical Cancer Research. 2020;**39**:24. DOI: 10.1186/s13046-020-1528-x

[27] Li H, Zhao B, Liu Y, Deng W, Zhang Y. Angiogenesis in residual cancer and roles of HIF-1α, VEGF, and MMP-9 in the development of residual cancer after radiofrequency ablation and surgical resection in rabbits with liver cancer. Folia Morphologica. 2020;**79**:71-78. DOI: 10.5603/FM.a2019.0059

[28] Tian QG, Wu YT, Liu Y, et al. Expressions and correlation analysis of HIF-1α, survivin and VEGF in patients with hepatocarcinoma. European Review for Medical and Pharmacological Sciences. 2018;**22**:3378-3385. DOI: 10.26355/eurrev_201806_15159

[29] Lin J, Cao S, Wang Y, et al. Long non-coding RNA UBE2CP3 enhances HCC cell secretion of VEGFA and promotes angiogenesis by activating ERK1/2/HIF-1α/VEGFA signalling in hepatocellular carcinoma. Journal of Experimental & Clinical Cancer Research. 2018;**37**:113. DOI: 10.1186/s13046-018-0727-1

[30] Damaghi M, Wojtkowiak JW, Gillies RJ. pH sensing and regulation in cancer. Frontiers in Physiology. 2013;**4**:370. DOI: 10.3389/fphys.2013.00370

[31] Nishi T, Forgac M. The vacuolar (H^+)-ATPases—Nature's most versatile proton pumps. Nature Reviews. Molecular Cell Biology. 2002;**3**:94-103. DOI:10.1038/nrm729

[32] Jefferies KC, Cipriano DJ, Forgac M. Function, structure and regulation of the vacuolar (H^+)-ATPases. Archives of Biochemistry and Biophysics. 2008;**476**:33-42. DOI: 10.1016/j.abb.2008.03.025

[33] Martinez-Zaguilan R, Lynch RM, Martinez GM, Gillies RJ. Vacuolar-type H(+)-ATPases are functionally expressed in plasma membranes of human tumor cells. The American Journal of Physiology. 1993;**265**:C1015-C1029. DOI: 10.1152/ajpcell.1993.265.4.C1015

[34] Sennoune SR, Bakunts K, Martínez GM, et al. Vacuolar H^+-ATPase in human breast cancer cells with distinct metastatic potential: Distribution and functional activity. American Journal of Physiology. Cell Physiology. 2004;**286**:C1443-C1452. DOI: 10.1152/ajpcell.00407.2003

[35] Fais S, De Milito A, You H, Qin W. Targeting vacuolar H^+-ATPases as a new strategy against cancer. Cancer Research. 2007;**67**:10627-10630. DOI: 10.1158/0008-5472.CAN-07-1805

[36] Xu J, Xie R, Liu X, et al. Expression and functional role of vacuolar H(+)-ATPase in human hepatocellular carcinoma. Carcinogenesis. 2012;**33**:2432-2440. DOI: 10.1093/carcin/bgs277

[37] Lu X, Chen L, Chen Y, Shao Q, Qin W. Bafilomycin A1 inhibits the growth and metastatic potential of the BEL-7402 liver cancer and HO-8910 ovarian cancer cell lines and induces alterations in their microRNA expression. Experimental and Therapeutic Medicine. 2015;**10**:1829-1834. DOI: 10.3892/etm.2015.2758

[38] Tang N, Jin J, Deng Y, et al. LASS2 interacts with V-ATPase and inhibits cell growth of hepatocellular carcinoma. Sheng Li Xue Bao. 2010;**62**:196-202 Chinese

[39] Li T, Tuo B. Pathophysiology of hepatic Na^+/H^+ exchange (review). Experimental and Therapeutic Medicine. 2020;**20**:1220-1229. DOI: 10.3892/etm.2020.8888

[40] Sardet C, Franchi A, Pouysségur J. Molecular cloning, primary structure, and expression of the human growth factor-activatable Na^+/H^+ antiporter. Cell. 1989;**56**:271-280. DOI: 10.1016/0092-8674(89)90901-x

[41] Yang X, Wang D, Dong W, Song Z, Dou K. Expression and modulation of Na(+)/H(+) exchanger 1 gene in hepatocellular carcinoma: A potential therapeutic target. Journal of Gastroenterology and Hepatology. 2011;**26**:364-370. DOI: 10.1111/j.1440-1746.2010.06382.x

[42] Kim SW, Cha MJ, Lee SK, et al. Curcumin treatment in combination with glucose restriction inhibits intracellular alkalinization and tumor growth in hepatoma cells. International Journal of Molecular Sciences. 2019;**20**:2375. DOI: 10.3390/ijms20102375

[43] Li X, Tsauo J, Geng C, Zhao H, Lei X, Li X. Ginsenoside Rg3 decreases NHE1 expression via inhibiting EGF-EGFR-ERK1/2-HIF-1 α pathway in hepatocellular carcinoma: A novel antitumor mechanism. The American Journal of Chinese Medicine. 2018;**46**:1915-1931. DOI: 10.1142/S0192415X18500969

[44] Payen VL, Mina E, Van Hée VF, Porporato PE, Sonveaux P. Monocarboxylate transporters in cancer. Molecular Metabolism. 2020;**33**:48-66. DOI: 10.1016/j.molmet.2019.07.006

[45] de la Cruz-López KG, Castro-Muñoz LJ, Reyes-Hernández DO, García-Carrancá A, Manzo-Merino J. Lactate in the regulation of tumor microenvironment and therapeutic approaches. Frontiers in Oncology. 2019;**9**:1143. DOI: 10.3389/fonc.2019.01143

[46] Alves VA, Pinheiro C, Morais-Santos F, Felipe-Silva A, Longatto-Filho A, Baltazar F. Characterization of monocarboxylate transporter activity in hepatocellular carcinoma. World Journal of Gastroenterology. 2014;**20**:11780-11787. DOI: 10.3748/wjg.v20.i33.11780

[47] Halestrap AP, Wilson MC. The monocarboxylate transporter family—Role and regulation. IUBMB Life. 2012;**64**:109-119. DOI: 10.1002/iub.572

[48] Chen HL, OuYang HY, Le Y, et al. Aberrant MCT4 and GLUT1 expression is correlated with early recurrence and poor prognosis of hepatocellular carcinoma after hepatectomy. Cancer Medicine. 2018;**7**:5339-5350. DOI: 10.1002/cam4.1521

[49] Nath K, Guo L, Nancolas B, et al. Mechanism of antineoplastic activity of lonidamine. Biochimica et Biophysica Acta. 2016;**1866**:151-162. DOI: 10.1016/j.bbcan.2016.08.001

[50] Waheed A, Sly WS. Carbonic anhydrase XII functions in health and disease. Gene. 2017;**623**:33-40. DOI: 10.1016/j.gene.2017.04.027

[51] Xing X, Yuan H, Liu H, et al. Quantitative secretome analysis reveals clinical values of carbonic anhydrase II in hepatocellular carcinoma. Genomics, Proteomics & Bioinformatics. 2021;**19**:94-107. DOI: 10.1016/j.gpb.2020.09.005

[52] Finkelmeier F, Canli Ö, Peiffer KH, et al. Circulating hypoxia marker carbonic anhydrase IX (CA9) in patients with hepatocellular carcinoma and patients with cirrhosis. PLoS One. 2018;**13**:e0200855. DOI: 10.1371/journal.pone.0200855

[53] Zeng X, Yin F, Liu X, et al. Upregulation of E2F transcription factor 3 is associated with poor prognosis in hepatocellular carcinoma. Oncology Reports. 2014;**31**:1139-1146. DOI: 10.3892/or.2014.2968

[54] Uda NR, Stenner F, Seibert V, et al. Humanized monoclonal antibody blocking carbonic anhydrase 12 enzymatic activity leads to reduced tumor growth in vitro. Anticancer Research. 2019;**39**:4117-4128. DOI: 10.21873/anticanres.13570

[55] Han R, Yang H, Lu L, Lin L. Tiliroside as a CAXII inhibitor suppresses liver cancer development and modulates E2Fs/Caspase-3 axis. Scientific Reports. 2021;**11**:8626. DOI: 10.1038/s41598-021-88133-7

[56] Carattino MD, Montalbetti N. Acid-sensing ion channels in sensory signaling. American Journal of Physiology. Renal Physiology. 2020;**318**:F531-F543. DOI: 10.1152/ajprenal.00546.2019

[57] Storozhuk M, Cherninskyi A, Maximyuk O, Isaev D, Krishtal O.

Acid-sensing ion channels: Focus on physiological and some pathological roles in the brain. Current Neuropharmacology. 2021;**19**: 1570-1589. DOI: 10.2174/ 1570159X19666210125151824

[58] Jin C, Yuan FL, Gu YL, et al. Over-expression of ASIC1a promotes proliferation via activation of the β-catenin/LEF-TCF axis and is associated with disease outcome in liver cancer. Oncotarget. 2017;**8**:25977-25988. DOI: 10.18632/oncotarget.10774

[59] Jin C, Zhu MQ, Yuan FL, et al. The expressions of acid sensing ion channel la and activator protein-1 in hepatocellular carcinoma and their relationships with clinical features. Chinese Journal of Hepatobiliary Surgery. 2018;**24**:376-380. DOI: 10.3760/ cma.j.issn.1007-8118.2018.06.005

[60] Bujak JK, Kosmala D, Szopa IM, Majchrzak K, Bednarczyk P. Inflammation, cancer and immunity-implication of TRPV1 channel. Frontiers in Oncology. 2019;**9**:1087. DOI: 10.3389/ fonc.2019.01087

[61] Miao X, Liu G, Xu X, et al. High expression of vanilloid receptor-1 is associated with better prognosis of patients with hepatocellular carcinoma. Cancer Genetics and Cytogenetics. 2008;**186**:25-32. DOI: 10.1016/j. cancergencyto.2008.05.011

[62] Xie C, Liu G, Li M, et al. Targeting TRPV1 on cellular plasticity regulated by Ovol 2 and Zeb 1 in hepatocellular carcinoma. Biomedicine & Pharmacotherapy. 2019;**118**:109270. DOI: 10.1016/j.biopha.2019.109270

[63] Scheau C, Badarau IA, Caruntu C, et al. Capsaicin: Effects on the pathogenesis of hepatocellular carcinoma. Molecules. 2019;**24**:2350. DOI: 10.3390/molecules24132350

[64] Wong MM, Chan HY, Aziz NA, et al. Interplay of autophagy and cancer stem cells in hepatocellular carcinoma. Molecular Biology Reports. 2021;**48**:3695-3717. DOI: 10.1007/ s11033-021-06334-9

[65] Li X, Li C, Zhang L, et al. The significance of exosomes in the development and treatment of hepatocellular carcinoma. Molecular Cancer. 2020;**19**:1. DOI: 10.1186/ s12943-019-1085-0

[66] Wang H, Lu Z, Zhao X. Tumorigenesis, diagnosis, and therapeutic potential of exosomes in liver cancer. Journal of Hematology & Oncology. 2019;**12**:133. DOI: 10.1186/ s13045-019-0806-6

[67] Liu Y, Shi K, Chen Y, et al. Exosomes and their role in cancer progression. Frontiers in Oncology. 2021;**11**:639159. DOI: 10.3389/fonc.2021.639159

[68] Panagiotou N, Neytchev O, Selman C, Shiels PG. Extracellular vesicles, ageing, and therapeutic interventions. Cell. 2018;**7**:110. DOI: 10.3390/cells7080110

[69] Tian XP, Wang CY, Jin XH, et al. Acidic microenvironment up-regulates exosomal miR-21 and miR-10b in early-stage hepatocellular carcinoma to promote cancer cell proliferation and metastasis. Theranostics. 2019;**9**:1965-1979. DOI: 10.7150/thno.30958

[70] Greening DW, Gopal SK, Mathias RA, et al. Emerging roles of exosomes during epithelial-mesenchymal transition and cancer progression. Seminars in Cell & Developmental Biology. 2015;**40**:60-71. DOI: 10.1016/j. semcdb.2015.02.008

[71] Meng X, Xu Y, Ning X. Tumor microenvironment acidity modulates

ROR1 to promote epithelial-mesenchymal transition and hepatocarcinoma metastasis. Journal of Cell Science. 2021;**134**:jcs255349. DOI: 10.1242/jcs.255349

[72] Takahashi K, Yan IK, Haga H, Patel T. Modulation of hypoxia-signaling pathways by extracellular linc-RoR. Journal of Cell Science. 2014;**127**:1585-1594. DOI: 10.1242/jcs.141069

[73] Ludwig N, Whiteside TL. Potential roles of tumor-derived exosomes in angiogenesis. Expert Opinion on Therapeutic Targets. 2018;**22**:409-417. DOI: 10.1080/14728222.2018.1464141

[74] Shao C, Yang F, Miao S, et al. Role of hypoxia-induced exosomes in tumor biology. Molecular Cancer. 2018;**17**:120. DOI: 10.1186/s12943-018-0869-y

[75] Lee TK, Poon RT, Yuen AP, et al. Regulation of angiogenesis by Id-1 through hypoxia-inducible factor-1alpha-mediated vascular endothelial growth factor up-regulation in hepatocellular carcinoma. Clinical Cancer Research. 2006;**12**:6910-6919. DOI: 10.1158/1078-0432.CCR-06-0489

[76] Song J, Ge Z, Yang X, et al. Hepatic stellate cells activated by acidic tumor microenvironment promote the metastasis of hepatocellular carcinoma via osteopontin. Cancer Letters. 2015;**356**:713-720. DOI: 10.1016/j.canlet.2014.10.021

[77] Wolchok JD, Neyns B, Linette G, et al. Ipilimumab monotherapy in patients with pretreated advanced melanoma: A randomised, double-blind, multicentre, phase 2, dose-ranging study. The Lancet Oncology. 2010;**11**:155-164. DOI: 10.1016/S1470-2045(09)70334-1

[78] Huber V, Camisaschi C, Berzi A, et al. Cancer acidity: An ultimate frontier of tumor immune escape and a novel target of immunomodulation. Seminars in Cancer Biology. 2017;**43**:74-89. DOI: 10.1016/j.semcancer.2017.03.001

[79] Veglia F, Sanseviero E, Gabrilovich DI. Myeloid-derived suppressor cells in the era of increasing myeloid cell diversity. Nature Reviews. Immunology. 2021;**21**(8):485-498. DOI: 10.1038/s41577-020-00490-y

[80] Labiano S, Palazon A, Melero I. Immune response regulation in the tumor microenvironment by hypoxia. Seminars in Oncology. 2015;**42**:378-386. DOI: 10.1053/j.seminoncol.2015.02.009

[81] Cubillos-Ruiz JR, Mohamed E, Rodriguez PC. Unfolding anti-tumor immunity: ER stress responses sculpt tolerogenic myeloid cells in cancer. Journal for Immunotherapy of Cancer. 2017;**5**:5. DOI: 10.1186/s40425-016-0203-4

[82] Chouaib S, Noman MZ, Kosmatopoulos K, Curran MA. Hypoxic stress: Obstacles and opportunities for innovative immunotherapy of cancer. Oncogene. 2017;**36**:439-445. DOI: 10.1038/onc.2016.225

[83] Egners A, Erdem M, Cramer T. The response of macrophages and neutrophils to hypoxia in the context of cancer and other inflammatory diseases. Mediators of Inflammation. 2016;**2016**:2053646. DOI: 10.1155/2016/2053646

[84] Chen J, Cao X, Li B, et al. Warburg effect is a cancer immune evasion mechanism against macrophage immunosurveillance. Frontiers in Immunology. 2021;**11**:621757. DOI: 10.3389/fimmu.2020.621757

[85] Lim AR, Rathmell WK, Rathmell JC. The tumor microenvironment as a metabolic barrier to effector T cells and

immunotherapy. eLife. 2020;**9**:e55185. DOI: 10.7554/eLife.55185

[86] Pötzl J, Roser D, Bankel L, et al. Reversal of tumor acidosis by systemic buffering reactivates NK cells to express IFN-γ and induces NK cell-dependent lymphoma control without other immunotherapies. International Journal of Cancer. 2017;**140**:2125-2133. DOI: 10.1002/ijc.30646

[87] Mollinedo F. Neutrophil degranulation, plasticity, and cancer metastasis. Trends in Immunology. 2019;**40**:228-242. DOI: 10.1016/j.it.2019.01.006

[88] Trevani AS, Andonegui G, Giordano M, et al. Extracellular acidification induces human neutrophil activation. Journal of Immunology. 1999;**162**:4849-4857

[89] Worsley CM, Veale RB, Mayne ES. The acidic tumour microenvironment: Manipulating the immune response to elicit escape. Human Immunology. 2022;**83**:399-408. DOI: 10.1016/j.humimm.2022.01.014

[90] Jiang P, Mizushima N. Autophagy and human diseases. Cell Research. 2014;**24**:69-79. DOI: 10.1038/cr.2013.161

[91] Ghavami S, Gupta S, Ambrose E, Hnatowich M, Freed DH, Dixon IM. Autophagy and heart disease: Implications for cardiac ischemia-reperfusion damage. Current Molecular Medicine. 2014; **14**:616-629. DOI: 10.2174/1566524014666140603101520

[92] Hashimoto D, Bläuer M, Hirota M, Ikonen NH, Sand J, Laukkarinen J. Autophagy is needed for the growth of pancreatic adenocarcinoma and has a cytoprotective effect against anticancer drugs. European Journal of Cancer. 2014;**50**:1382-1390. DOI: 10.1016/j.ejca.2014.01.011

[93] Ryter SW, Choi AM. Autophagy in lung disease pathogenesis and therapeutics. Redox Biology. 2015;**4**:215-225. DOI: 10.1016/j.redox.2014.12.010

[94] Chao X, Qian H, Wang S, Fulte S, Ding WX. Autophagy and liver cancer. Clinical and Molecular Hepatology. 2020;**26**:606-617. DOI: 10.3350/cmh.2020.0169

[95] Fan Q, Yang L, Zhang X, et al. Autophagy promotes metastasis and glycolysis by upregulating MCT1 expression and Wnt/β-catenin signaling pathway activation in hepatocellular carcinoma cells. Journal of Experimental & Clinical Cancer Research. 2018;**37**:9. DOI: 10.1186/s13046-018-0673-y

[96] Jiao L, Zhang HL, Li DD, et al. Regulation of glycolytic metabolism by autophagy in liver cancer involves selective autophagic degradation of HK2 (hexokinase 2). Autophagy. 2018;**14**:671-684. DOI: 10.1080/15548627.2017.1381804

[97] Wang S, Lv Y, Zhou Y, et al. Acidic extracellular pH induces autophagy to promote anoikis resistance of hepatocellular carcinoma cells via downregulation of miR-3663-3p. Journal of Cancer. 2021;**12**:3418-3426. DOI: 10.7150/jca.51849

[98] Forner A, Reig M, Bruix J. Hepatocellular carcinoma. Lancet. 2018;**391**:1301-1314. DOI: 10.1016/S0140-6736(18)30010-2

[99] Llovet JM, Ricci S, Mazzaferro V, et al. Sorafenib in advanced hepatocellular carcinoma. The New England Journal of Medicine. 2008;**359**:378-390. DOI: 10.1056/NEJMoa0708857

[100] Tang W, Chen Z, Zhang W, et al. The mechanisms of sorafenib resistance in hepatocellular carcinoma: Theoretical basis and therapeutic aspects. Signal Transduction and Targeted

Therapy. 2020;**5**:87. DOI: 10.1038/s41392-020-0187-x

[101] Colagrande S, Regini F, Taliani GG, Nardi C, Inghilesi AL. Advanced hepatocellular carcinoma and sorafenib: Diagnosis, indications, clinical and radiological follow-up. World Journal of Hepatology. 2015;7:1041-1053. DOI: 10.4254/wjh.v7.i8.1041

[102] Liu LP, Ho RL, Chen GG, Lai PB. Sorafenib inhibits hypoxia-inducible factor-1α synthesis: Implications for antiangiogenic activity in hepatocellular carcinoma. Clinical Cancer Research. 2012;**18**:5662-5671. DOI: 10.1158/1078-0432.CCR-12-0552

[103] Xu M, Xie XH, Xie XY, et al. Sorafenib suppresses the rapid progress of hepatocellular carcinoma after insufficient radiofrequency ablation therapy: An experiment in vivo. Acta Radiologica. 2013;**54**:199-204. DOI: 10.1258/ar.2012.120249

[104] Liang Y, Zheng T, Song R, et al. Hypoxia-mediated sorafenib resistance can be overcome by EF24 through Von Hippel-Lindau tumor suppressor-dependent HIF-1α inhibition in hepatocellular carcinoma. Hepatology. 2013;**57**:1847-1857. DOI: 10.1002/hep.26224

[105] Pilon-Thomas S, Kodumudi KN, El-Kenawi AE, et al. Neutralization of tumor acidity improves antitumor responses to immunotherapy. Cancer Research. 2016;**76**:1381-1390. DOI: 10.1158/0008-5472.CAN-15-1743

[106] Fais S, Marunaka Y. The acidic microenvironment: Is it a phenotype of all cancers? A focus on multiple myeloma and some analogies with diabetes mellitus. Cancers (Basel). 2020;**12**:3226. DOI: 10.3390/cancers12113226

[107] Bhattacharya B, Low SH, Soh C, et al. Increased drug resistance is associated with reduced glucose levels and an enhanced glycolysis phenotype. British Journal of Pharmacology. 2014;**171**:3255-3267. DOI: 10.1111/bph.12668

[108] Wong WY, DeLuca CI, Tian B, et al. Urease-induced alkalinization of extracellular pH and its antitumor activity in human breast and lung cancers. Journal of Experimental Therapeutics & Oncology. 2005;**5**:93-99

[109] Bhattacharya B, Huang DQ, Low SHH, et al. Effect of cell microenvironment on the drug sensitivity of hepatocellular cancer cells. Oncotarget. 2021;**12**:674-685. DOI: 10.18632/oncotarget.27910

[110] Bergers G, Fendt SM. The metabolism of cancer cells during metastasis. Nature Reviews. Cancer. 2021;**21**:162-180. DOI: 10.1038/s41568-020-00320-2

[111] Piñero F, Dirchwolf M, Pessôa MG. Biomarkers in hepatocellular carcinoma: Diagnosis, prognosis and treatment response assessment. Cells. 2020;**9**:1370. DOI: 10.3390/cells9061370

[112] Kremer M, Manzini G, Hartel M. Lebermetastasen: aktueller Stand der chirurgischen Behandlungsmöglichkeiten [Current surgical treatment options for liver metastasis]. Therapeutische Umschau. 2021;**78**:597-603. DOI: 10.1024/0040-5930/a001316

[113] Li YM, Wei YC. Reconsideration of surgical treatment for liver cancer. Zhonghua Yi Xue Za Zhi. 2021;**101**:2179-2184. DOI: 10.3760/cma.j.cn112137-20210411-00865

[114] Song TQ. Changes and challenges of surgical treatment strategy for hepatocellular carcinoma. Zhong hua Wai Ke Za Zhi. 2021;**59**:447-451. DOI:10.3760/cma.j.cn112139-20201209-00849